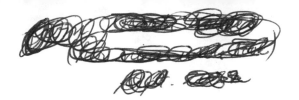

The Body Tune-Up:
A Food-Based
Cleanse

6 weeks to lifelong
healthy habits

Katy Wallace, ND

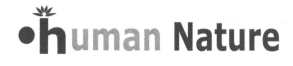

ISBN 978-1-957077-15-4

Portrait photography on back cover by Eric Tadsen

Interior black-and-white illustrations copyright © 2021 by Marian Wallace

The information in this book is for health education purposes only and not intended as a substitute for the advice and care of your physician. As with all new nutrition programs, the health and wellness program should be followed only after consulting with your physician to make sure it is right for you. Nutritional needs vary from person to person. The author and publisher expressly disclaim responsibility for any adverse effects that may result from the use or application of the information contained in this book.

Publisher's Cataloging-in-Publication data

Names: Wallace, Katy, author.
Title: The body tune-up : a food-based cleanse, 6 weeks to lifelong healthy habits / Katy Wallace, ND.
Description: Includes bibliographical references. | Madison, WI: Katy Wallace, Human Nature, LLC, 2022.
Identifiers: ISBN: 978-1-957077-15-4
Subjects: LCSH Detoxification (Health) | Self-care, Health.| BISAC HEALTH & FITNESS / Body Cleansing & Detoxification | HEALTH & FITNESS / Naturopathy | HEALTH & FITNESS / Diet & Nutrition / General
Classification: LCC RA784.5 W35 2022 | DDC 613--dc23

Table of Contents

Preface

Working as a naturopath for fourteen years, I have seen the amazing transformations people experience using a food-based approach. In the beginning of my career, my focus was guiding people through food-based cleanses and making cleanses more accessible and understandable. After this period, I began to see limitations and potential drawbacks of cleansing. I turned to professional trainings in functional medicine to identify ways to help someone whose health problems were not easily resolved by food-based cleansing, or who were not able to cleanse. Today, I share this combination of healing through food and functional medicine as the basis of my practice. I approach food-based cleansing gently, with a scientific approach.

Despite the language used, the ultimate long-term goal of the food-based approach outlined in this book is not to "cleanse." The goal is to provide your body with much-needed nourishment and assist your innate ability to rejuvenate from within. Yes, this process can include releasing unwanted waste and toxins and old habits that are not serving your highest good. However, it is my hope your experience with food-based cleansing will be just a stepping-stone to better support your health through nutrient-dense foods in daily meals for the rest of your life.

My path to this creative and science-based way of working with people did not come easily. I underwent my first food-based cleanse when I was twenty-six years old. I was working as an ecological scientist in southern Wisconsin, a couple years out of graduate school, and I had fatigue and was sick. Every several weeks, I would come down with a virus that would become a sinus infection. I would get antibiotics from the doctor and feel better for about two weeks, and then the cycle would start all over again. I had been told I was healthy by medical doctors who did not have much time to talk with me and said I needed another dose of antibiotics. This had been going on for over a year when a friend and colleague suggested I pay a visit to her naturopath, Dr. Renee Welhouse. Other friends had been encouraging me to find a naturopath too, so I was ready to check it out.

I made my first visit to Dr. Renee at the Welhouse Center in the fall of 2003. I was surprised when she told me the issue was my gut and she had a plan to help me get better. Despite the newness of the ideas she shared, I felt relieved that someone believed me that something was wrong and knew how to help.

I left Dr. Renee's office with a bag full of supplements including green drink powder, vitamins, and a digestive cleanse kit. At home, I told my fiancé, Woody, that I was going to do what she said: for the next eleven days, I would eat acid fruits for breakfast and low-starch vegetables and fats for lunch and dinner. Woody was skeptical but could see that I was committed to trying this, so he made me a large stir-fry of ginger with asparagus for dinner. I ate Granny Smith apples in the morning. I remember being a little hungry toting my asparagus leftovers around in my backpack while doing fieldwork in Chicago-area wetlands for work. I hated the green drink and didn't take it until several weeks later.

I unknowingly blew the cleanse one day when we had guests visiting from out of town who wanted to watch a movie. I convinced myself popcorn was a vegetable and could be had on the cleanse. I promptly took a nap from the starch overload. It wasn't the perfect cleanse, but I did start to feel something changing for the better, so I went back to see Dr. Renee.

Over the next several months, she suggested I do multiple cleanses, including parasite, kidney, and liver cleanses, as well as colonics. Yes, I saw the evidence of the cleansing in the toilet (a tapeworm I had picked up working in the rain forest in Maui and small green balls from my gallbladder at the culmination of the gallbladder flush). The day she told me to do a ten-day water fast, I cried in her office at the thought of being restricted in the ultimate sense. She ignored that I was crying and told me to get started. After the ten-day fast, there was an SOS cleanse that included drinking sodium sulfate salts and fasting on fresh juice and receiving body work, Chi Machine, steam baths, and more.

Ultimately, I ended up feeling much better, experienced no sinus infections, and learned a new way of eating. Fast-forward a couple years and I decided to make a career change and go back to school to become a naturopath and nutritionist myself. Today, eighteen years following that first cleanse, I can say I have helped thousands of people through food-based cleanses.

Dr. Renee's approach to food-based cleansing was intense, but it generally offered positive and almost immediate results. She herself had started cleansing to save her own life and the lives of many clients from cancer. I found the cleanse to be a way to get back in touch with my body and how I cared for it in a way no one had ever discussed with me. I eventually left the field of ecology and worked as a nutritionist and office manager under Dr. Renee while I worked toward my naturopathic doctor degree (ND). When I was ready to start my own business, Human Nature, LLC, I started teaching food-based cleansing in a group workshop format known as "The Body Tune-Up." I felt driven to share this information that had made a profound change for me and others.

Over the years, I have adapted the Body Tune-Up to be a gentler process than the cleansing plan I learned from Dr. Renee. For example, knowing that most people experience chronic stress or overtaxed adrenals and thyroid, I include more protein in the plan and leave out the ten-day water fast at the end. Knowing that many people suffer from blood sugar dysfunction, I have minimized fruit. Eighteen years ago, we didn't know that whole grains exacerbate leaky gut and inflammation, but now we do, so these foods are avoided. There are many ways the Body Tune-Up may be adapted to the individual, and I encourage you to be self-aware and make adaptations where needed. However, be prepared that you might not get the results you are seeking unless you stay true to the suggestions in the book.

As of spring 2021, our office has offered fourteen annual Body Tune-Up workshops. Even though cleansing has been around for a while and the "fad" of it comes and goes, I still find that cleansing has immense value for people. For many, cleansing allows a finite period during which they can devote themselves to rebooting their food routine and health. While this workshop has traditionally been offered in a group format in person, we now offer individual and group consultation in virtual settings. If you would like to learn more about how we can support you in your health journey, you can find our contact information in Appendix C of this book. It is my pleasure to bring what I've learned from Dr. Renee and my experience leading the cleanses to a wider audience through this book. I hope you receive many lifelong benefits from your experience with it.

Katy Wallace, ND
Madison, WI

Part 1: Introduction & Preparation

Chapter 1: Food-Based Cleansing

Food-based cleansing is the process of eating specific foods to promote health and rejuvenation in the body. This book is designed to outline cleansing protocols that support the body's natural ability to detoxify and obtain optimal health through food.

During a food-based cleanse, you avoid foods that may be stressful to your body. A specific list of foods to eat is provided for each cleanse to achieve a healthier outcome. A food-based cleanse may allow for the reintroduction of foods gradually over time. In this way, it can also serve as an elimination period where you may "test" the response of your body to the reintroduction of foods with the aim of sustaining a healthy food plan for you.

This Body Tune-Up workshop takes you through four consecutive cleanses: the Digestive Cleanse, Critter Cleanse, Kidney Cleanse, and Liver Cleanse. Each protocol combines a special food plan with supplements that support the aim of each cleanse.

Foods that may cause inflammation are avoided, and foods that provide nutrients to promote detoxification are encouraged. In this way, the special food plan supports the body by providing nutrients required for health. Throughout the book, I reference supplements and tools that can help assist the health and cleansing of the body. Suggestions for how to access these items are included in Appendix C.

What does a food-based cleanse do for my body?

1) Normalize blood sugar levels and balance insulin.

We avoid foods containing natural sugars, like fruits and sweeteners, to allow insulin levels to normalize and reverse the inflammatory impact of insulin in the body. Insulin production drives many illnesses, including metabolic syndrome, hormone imbalances, and low energy. Reducing foods that contain appreciable carbohydrates also helps with the utilization of vitamins like vitamin C inside the body's cells. Balanced insulin levels help improve brain and neurotransmitter performance as well.

2) Repair the gut lining.

We avoid foods that tend to aggravate the gut lining and cause increased intestinal permeability, like whole grains (even quinoa) and legumes. Improving the health of the gut lining is key to resolving many chronic problems, including food sensitivities, autoimmunity, hormonal and blood sugar issues, mood problems, and immune stress. We emphasize foods and supplements that encourage the growth of beneficial organisms.

3) Reduce a negative immune response.

Foods with a large molecular peptide structure (like gluten, dairy, and gums like carrageenan) tend to become a target for the immune system, leading to the release of immune chemicals called cytokines that perpetuate pain and chronic inflammation. Eating these foods can make it harder to heal or have optimum health. Modulating the immune system, or being able to modify and control it, is key to overcoming chronic inflammation and disease, especially autoimmune diseases. Therefore, we avoid the foods that we know from clinical research and experience tend to aggravate the immune system, making modulation more difficult. Through specific foods and supplements, the immune system and glandular system are able to function more healthfully.

In addition, decreased inflammation for the nervous system leads to mental and emotional benefits.

4) Provide key nutrients that assist with detoxification.
Our bodies are exposed to toxins every day, including heavy metals, pesticides, plastics, industrial and medical chemicals, and bacterial endotoxins (which result from poor digestion and leaky gut and lead to inflammation). In some cases, toxins are not eliminated efficiently and can accumulate in tissues and organs. If your detoxification pathways are not as strong as they should be, you can even become toxic from food, drink, body care products, and environmental allergens. The accumulation of toxins disrupts healthy cell function and increases the risk for disease. Improper removal of toxins over time can lead to poor health. When toxins enter our cells, the body has three steps or "phases" of detoxification. Proper nutrition helps ensure that each step is supported. This is one of the reasons for the Body Tune-Up's emphasis on food specifications both during and after the cleanses.

It is also critical to establish and maintain a healthy gut biome. Many of the dysfunctions already mentioned (blood sugar imbalance, leaky gut, negative immune response, lack of detoxification) originate from an imbalance in the bacteria of the gut, known as the gut flora or biome. When the gut is out of balance, toxins (either innate or manmade) may more easily circulate through the body and create unwanted symptoms. Providing your cells with an upgrade in nutrients can improve the cellular health of any part of the body.

It can be helpful when cleansing to use a "binder," something that attracts the toxin and helps the body eliminate it in a bowel movement. Digestive enzymes and probiotics may be helpful in reestablishing healthy digestion and healthy gut flora. In the Critter Cleanse, herbs and supplements are used to reduce overgrowths of unwanted organisms.

What ailments can a cleanse help with?
People have undergone food-based cleansing to address ailments like digestive distress, chronic fatigue, weight loss resistance, brain fog, migraines, sinus infections, food sensitivities, painful joints, depleted

energy, anxiety, hot flashes, lung problems, increased risk for heart disease, and others.

What can I expect from a cleanse?

People can expect varying outcomes through different phases of the cleanse. Generally, the longer one adheres to a healthy food plan, the greater the benefits. The hope is that this six-week period will be an introduction to a long-term improvement.

It is common for people, as they undergo the Digestive Cleanse phase, to find it easier to wake up in the morning and feel lighter throughout the day. They do not have large fluctuations in energy before or after meals but instead have steady energy.

During the first phase of the cleanse—the Digestive Cleanse—it is common to be hungrier during the first few days as the body moves from getting its calories from quick-burning carbs to slower-metabolizing meat, fat, and vegetables. This very low carb way of eating is also referred to as a ketogenic food plan, named for the ketones produced when the liver burns fat for energy. Ketones are a powerful energy source for the body, especially for the brain and muscles. Most people report a greater sense of satiation on the ketogenic food plan (due to fat burning) and greater energy and mental clarity. To ensure sustained energy throughout the day, it is helpful to keep cleanse-friendly snacks on hand. Some people adopt a ketogenic food plan long term due to its health benefits.

In this book, only the Digestive Cleanse food program typically brings about ketone production for the average person. Ketones have a diuretic effect, which means excess water is lost through increased urination. It is not uncommon for people to lose several pounds of water weight as they shift from insulin production to fat-burning mode or stop eating a food like bread that is inflammatory for them. It is important to drink plenty of fluids for you to feel good through this phase.

At the end of the Digestive Cleanse, a person may continue the ketogenic food plan by not adding in starchy vegetables and fruits that are otherwise suggested for the Critter Cleanse.

As the cleanse progresses, it is common for participants to experience reduced food cravings, improved sleep, normalized bowel movements, reduced gas and bloating, decreased pain levels, and increased mental clarity.

The Body Tune-Up can be instrumental for those experiencing weight loss resistance. Numerous people have been able to lose weight doing the Tune-Up when nothing else had worked for them. This is due to a combination of the characteristics of the process:

- It promotes a reduction in inflammation, which then makes it easier to lose weight.
- It improves blood sugar control, which helps better regulate the hormone cortisol and thus help with weight loss.
- It promotes fat-burning and thus weight loss.
- It supports a healthy metabolism through the inclusion of protein-rich, fat-dense foods and low-starch vegetables.

For example, one participant suffered from high levels of stress, and food sensitivities, and despite following many special diets, she had been unsuccessful in losing weight. With the Body Tune-Up, she experienced a newfound calm with the magnesium baths and was successful in losing over twenty pounds and keeping it off.

Chapter 2: Overview of Organ Cleanses

Week Prior to the Cleanse (4–7 Days before the Cleanse Starts)

If you are not used to clean eating, begin to decrease your daily intake of less healthy foods prior to the official Day 1 of the Digestive Cleanse, including coffee and caffeinated drinks, white bread and pastas, processed foods, fried foods, sweets, alcohol, and nicotine. Increase your vegetable and water intake.

Take some time for yourself and identify your goals for the cleanse. Build a support network for yourself with family and friends. Try to keep social and work engagements to a minimum during the cleanse. Make a few of the suggested recipes and teas. As you will ideally be eating all home-cooked meals, you may want to precook some meals and freeze them. Some people prefer to wash, chop, and package their produce as soon as they get home from the market or store. You may find this saves you time or hassle later in the week.

Digestive Cleanse (10 Days)

This first period of cleansing is the Digestive Cleanse, which lasts ten days. This phase establishes the foundational plan of foods that cleanse and lubricate (mostly vegetables, fats, and optional protein). Recipes and a menu plan are included in this book. You may need to make a couple of trips to the farmers' market or grocery store, as you will be eating a lot of fresh produce. You will need to set aside more time to cook for yourself and organize snacks. Water, herbal teas, and green drinks are valuable during this time. You might choose to include supportive supplements that can enhance the cleanse, but the basis of the cleanse is food. *Digestive Cleanse details are in Chapter 7.*

Critter Cleanse (14–21 Days)

You have done the intense work of building your foundational food plan during the ten-day Digestive Cleanse and will now add in more of the supportive foods during the Critter Cleanse. This parasite cleanse consists of taking specific supplements and slowly adding additional healthful foods back into meals. As you add in new foods, try to space them at least one day apart so you can tell if you have a reaction to something. You could space new food introductions up to three or four days apart, as a food sensitivity might manifest over seventy-two hours in response. Green drinks and foods like chlorophyll and spirulina will help your body to detox any bad food reactions. Homemade soups, broths, and vegetables will be very beneficial. Natural health supplements like Ion* Biome and digestive enzymes can help with overcoming leaky gut in a case where a person has a number of food sensitivities. *Critter Cleanse details are in Chapter 8.*

Kidney Cleanse (4 Days)

You will mainly follow the food plan from the Critter Cleanse, with a few modifications. You will need to avoid additional diuretics like large amounts of herbal tea. You will be making a special tea and taking specific vitamins and herbs to support the kidneys. *Kidney Cleanse details are in Chapter 9.*

Liver Cleanse (12–13 Days)

After the Kidney Cleanse, you will take herbs for the liver in the form of tablets called Body Tune-Up Liver Support, which may be chewed or swallowed whole. You will continue to eat a proper food combining plan including plenty of foods that benefit the liver. After ten days of the tablets, you will have two "apple days," followed by a cleansing cocktail. If you have blood sugar issues, you may eat vegetables instead of apples.

Do not add in too many new foods too quickly after the Liver Cleanse so you can better gauge the effects of new foods as they are "tested." Breads and baked goods, processed foods, coffee, sugar, and alcohol are examples of foods that may sabotage the benefits you have gained from cleaning up your food plan, so plan to avoid these for a while. *Liver Cleanse details are in Chapter 10.*

Testing Period after the Cleanse (30+ Days)

At this point, you've developed a foundational food plan over the previous six weeks and have eliminated the highly reactive foods. You now have a chance to test foods you are reintroducing to see if you are sensitive to them. If you think you have a reaction to a certain food, avoid that food for at least another six weeks, and then you could try it again.

Ideally, you will continue to avoid caffeinated drinks, fried foods, sugar, flour products, and sweets in the long term for continued optimal health.

Many of the supplements mentioned throughout this book can be purchased through Human Nature, LLC. Please see Appendix C for more information on how to get them.

Chapter 3: The Process of Cleansing

In the process of cleansing, you may experience some discomfort as your body adjusts.

First, your body may have a hard time digesting new food it is not used to. For example, if you do not typically eat a lot of vegetables, fat, or animal protein, this may be an adjustment for your body. Slowly phasing in new foods a few days before you officially start can help with this. A digestive enzyme taken each time you eat can also help.

Second, your insulin and other hormone levels may be adjusting as you switch from carb-burning to fat-burning energy production during the cleanse. Ultimately, this will give you better energy and mental clarity and help with reaching your optimal weight if this is an issue. This initial adjustment phase can make you feel tired but usually only lasts one to three days and then you feel better. Increasing your water and electrolyte intake and resting during this phase may help.

Lastly, all of us have some toxins in our bodies stored in our fat cells. When we shift to a healthy food plan and lifestyle, the stored toxins come out of the fat cells. Toxins in our cells flow into the extracellular fluid and are diffused into the bloodstream and then to the liver, kidneys, gastrointestinal tract, and skin systems as they are eliminated. Before the noxious substances are eliminated, these irritants often register in our body as side effects such as a headache, skin rashes/pimples, odoriferous stool and urine, decreased energy, and general malaise. Some people may have a more difficult time with this process of biotransformation also known as detoxification. Engaging in a cleanse is not foolproof. You may want to work with an experienced natural health care practitioner who can help you test or gauge how toxic your system is so you know what to expect from the cleanse. This is why in the group Body Tune-Up workshop, I meet privately with individual participants. This way I can better individualize a cleanse for them and offer more support where needed.

Think of healing side effects as an opportunity to resolve things that have not previously been resolved in your life, such as an injury (physical or emotional). A healing reaction may feel like the old condition, emotional trauma, or toxic treatment but in a diminished form. A crisis may last for a few days or even weeks. It is very important to give your body extra nutrition and extra support to assist in processing. The following section discusses supportive products and practices to help you during your cleanse.

Many people are surprised at how the Body Tune-Up helps with pain reduction. A twenty-nine-year-old man and his spouse did the Tune-Up together. They were newlyweds and loved to ballroom dance multiple hours two to three times weekly. The husband had complained that he had an injured knee that was keeping him from enjoying dancing, and he was concerned he would have to stop. Through the course of the Body Tune-Up, he reported having more energy and was able to increase his dancing due to the reduction in pain.

Chapter 4:
Detoxification: Kidney
& Liver Cleanses

Our bodies are exposed every day to toxins, which include heavy metals, pesticides, plastics, industrial chemicals, and bacterial endotoxins (which result from poor digestion and leaky gut and lead to inflammation). In some cases, toxins are not eliminated efficiently and can accumulate in tissues and organs. If your detoxification pathways are not as strong as they should be, you can even become toxic from things like food, drink, body care products, and environmental allergens. The accumulation of toxins disrupts healthy cell function and increases the risk for disease. Improper removal of toxins over time can lead to:

- obesity
- cardiovascular disease
- neurological and cognitive issues
- immune system dysfunction
- chemical intolerance
- reproductive and developmental concerns

Reducing the buildup of toxins internally is key to optimal health and longevity. The Kidney and Liver Cleanses support the innate ability of the body to detoxify.

When toxins enter our cells, the body has three steps or "phases" of detoxification. These steps need to work simultaneously in order for the detoxification to work effectively. Proper nutrition helps ensure that each step is supported. This is one of the reasons why I put a large emphasis on what you are eating during the Body Tune-Up. You need to be eating the right way to support the multiple phases of detoxification. The three phases of detoxification are activation, neutralization, and elimination.

Phase 1: Activation

Activation, or Phase 1, is when special enzymes form a reactive site to a toxin within the liver cells so that the body can better eliminate the toxin. Special nutrients in cruciferous vegetables (like broccoli and cabbage) and black radishes combine with an enzyme called myrosinase (high in foods like broccoli sprouts, mustard seeds, and horseradish) to get the toxin ready for the next step, Phase 2. In many cases, Phase 1 turns the toxin into something temporarily even more toxic so that it can be used in the next phase. Therefore, it is very important that Phase 2 be ready and well supported. Certain medicines and foods tend to upregulate Phase 1 without supporting Phase 2, and this is where some people can experience side effects from alcohol, chemicals, caffeine, sleeping pills, pesticides, prescription medications, et cetera.

Phase 2: Neutralization

Neutralization, or Phase 2, is the process of putting a protective compound (called conjugation) with the toxin so that it becomes less toxic and water soluble in order to be eliminated (sent from the liver via blood to the kidneys or via bile to the bowel to be excreted). Amino acids like glycine (found in high-protein foods like meat, fish, and legumes), antioxidants like glutathione, and substances like creatine (found in meats) that provide energy help to neutralize the toxin and get it ready for the next phase, elimination. Sulfur-rich foods are very important as well: onions, eggs, meats, garlic, cruciferous vegetables.

Phase 2 tends to be sluggish for some people. It is very important that Phase 2 be working, since Phase 1 metabolites can be dangerous and need to be moved out! For example, you might activate Phase 1 with your morning coffee and your evening wine. If you have a sluggish Phase 2, you will have symptoms of toxicity later, such as brain fog, insomnia, or hot flashes. Phase 2 requires the flow of bile, which helps eliminate the now-altered toxins from the liver and move them on to the bowel for elimination.

Phase 3: Elimination

Elimination, or Phase 3, is the final step in detoxification. This is where toxins are moved out of the body primarily through urine, feces, or sweat. Generally, having plenty of fats and alkaline-forming foods, as well as fiber, helps ensure the elimination phase is effective. Being properly hydrated is also important. A good supply of magnesium in the food plan and in food-based or chelated supplements is also important for elimination.

If there is a "bottleneck" in the system of toxin removal, then a person could be living with unnecessary symptoms and baggage. In order to resolve chronic health issues, it's important to make sure you receive enough support for daily detoxification. It can also be very helpful for people to undergo special periods of cleansing or detoxification, like the Kidney and Liver Cleanses. Remember, no cleanse is effective unless the digestive system is working effectively, so proper foods play a huge role in laying the groundwork for effective detoxification.

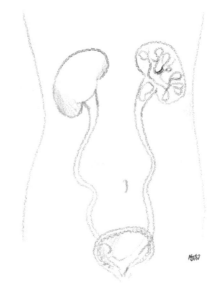

After the Digestive and Critter Cleanse, I focus on elimination through the kidneys, which filter the blood. The kidneys receive waste from the blood throughout the body, as well as the end products of detoxification from the liver. Therefore, I address the kidneys first to ensure they can handle the extra push resulting from the Liver Cleanse. I do this primarily with herbs and special foods like cherries that promote increased kidney filtering of the blood. The Kidney Cleanse is four days in duration.

The kidneys are a part of the urinary system that is a filtering center in the body. This includes the kidneys, the ureters, and the bladder. Kidneys are bean-shaped organs about the size of your fist. Each kidney contains about one million tiny filter units. Blood moves from the renal artery into the kidneys. Water, salts, toxic chemicals, excess minerals, waste, and urea (a waste product from the liver) are filtered by the kidneys. Salt and water needed by the body are reabsorbed into the renal vein and kept in the body. Waste products and surplus water leave through the ureters to the bladder. Healthy kidneys depend on good hydration, deep breathing, regular exercise, and a healthy food plan.

After the Kidney Cleanse, I suggest a Liver Cleanse. The Liver Cleanse includes herbs and special foods in a protocol that promotes the elimination of toxins from the liver and gallbladder. Besides its role in detoxification, the liver also has many other functions in the body. It helps regulate blood sugar by converting excess glucose into glycogen, the body's main source of stored energy. The liver also helps to modify hormones and inactivate them. The liver metabolizes and inactivates

A fifty-year-old woman, with the agreement of her doctor, took the Body Tune-Up workshop because she had high cholesterol and wanted to address it naturally. At the end of the cleanse, about four weeks after the Liver Cleanse, she was very pleased that her total cholesterol had dropped eighty points, enough for her to avoid needing to take cholesterol-lowering medications. By supporting the digestive system and liver, which allow for clearing old cholesterol, the Body Tune-Up can potentially help lower cholesterol. The food plan also helps reduce excess triglycerides and small-particle LDL cholesterol due to the reduction in processed carbohydrates.

both testosterone and estrogen. Therefore, when the liver is congested, proper hormone balance does not occur.

The liver metabolizes carbohydrates, proteins, and fats. If you have an overwhelmed liver, then you cannot utilize food as well, and you may have difficulty with different foods. The liver plays an intimate role in the absorption and storage of fat and fat-soluble vitamins from foods. It secretes bile, which is a bitter alkaline substance that is stored in the gallbladder and helps you to digest your fats (and the fat-soluble vitamins).

If you have trouble digesting fat, it is likely due to the gallbladder and liver needing more support. It is the liver's job to make bile—one to one and a half quarts daily! The liver is full of tubes that deliver the bile to the common bile duct, which is attached to the gallbladder and acts as a storage reservoir. Eating fat or protein triggers the gallbladder to squeeze itself empty after about twenty minutes. Bile then makes its way down to the small intestine. The bile helps emulsify the fats and lipase enzymes made in the pancreas to help absorb fat. The liver has thousands of biliary tubes inside it that can get clogged up. This causes a backup of bile and other liver products. Therefore, we do not get these helpful products in our digestive tract for digestion and elimination.

Also, we do not optimally clean or detoxify the blood without adequate bile flow. When you do the Liver Cleanse, you may pass extra bile in a few bowel movements. It may appear as small green pea-shaped globules, or perhaps darker "stones." There can be hard, calcified gallstones and also softer versions indicative of simply sluggish bile. The Liver Cleanse helps with detoxification and in relieving stagnation in the liver related to the liver's other functions.

Disclaimer: Carefully consider before engaging with the Kidney and Liver Cleanses if you are taking multiple medications, just to be safe. At least discuss it with your prescribing doctor before engaging in a kidney and liver detox program.

Glutathione: An Amazing Antioxidant

Do you know what the most abundant and important antioxidant in your body is? It is a molecule called glutathione (if we are excluding fresh water, which can also be a powerful antioxidant). Glutathione helps every cell in your body to detoxify. Our bodies synthesize glutathione from key amino acids, so it is important to eat and digest quality proteins such as grass-fed and wild animal products to make it. Glutathione provides several antioxidant processes in the body, including the following:

* **Detoxifying heavy metals and chemicals.** Glutathione helps your body turn harmful chemicals and metals into water-soluble chemicals to be excreted. Over time, glutathione levels in the body can be depleted by exposure to toxins. If someone is exposed to lead or mercury, for example, liposomal glutathione will help detoxify and eliminate the metals.

* **Addressing autoimmunity and inflammation.** Glutathione can play a big role in calming inflammation and autoimmunity via numerous pathways in the immune system. To help quickly get ahead of autoimmune activity, a supplement form of glutathione may be taken daily in conjunction with the Body Tune-Up protocol.

* **Helping overcome allergies and strong immune reactions.** Along the lines of immune modulation, glutathione can be taken to address histamine and mucus production in response to foods and other environmental triggers. This can work for chronic skin issues and common allergy signs. When my youngest daughter was four years old, she suffered from chronic sinus issues, which were complicating her preparation for a surgery she needed to repair the submucosal cleft palate. A doctor proposed steroids to get the sinus drainage under better control, since they could not find any medical reason for the sinus issues. As an alternative to steroids, I gave her Tri-fortify Orange, by Researched Nutritionals, and Turmero (an orange-flavored liquid turmeric extract), by Apex Energetics. Within days, her sinus congestion had cleared and she was ready for surgery, without the use of steroids and without side effects. The immune-modulating effects of glutathione and turmeric helped reduce her

congestion. We were also able to do an elimination period and identify that grains (including gluten-free ones) were the main trigger for her. This has helped to reduce allergies and sinus issues going forward.

* Maintaining a healthy gut lining and repairing leaky gut. *A reduction in glutathione is a key step in the development of leaky gut and autoimmune disease, according to recent studies. This antioxidant can be very powerful in protecting the body against these unwanted outcomes.*

* Protecting against fatigue. *All the above functions translate to an increase in energy, resilience to stress, greater athletic performance, strengthened immunity, reduction in inflammation, and slowing of the aging process. Liposomal glutathione can be a helpful support for the adrenals, thyroid, and pituitary. It has also been shown in studies to support weight loss.*

* Keeping other antioxidants active. *Glutathione helps maintain active forms of other antioxidants in the body, like vitamins C and E.*

* Lowering free-radical activity. *Neutralizes and/or regulates numerous oxidizing compounds in the body, such as hydrogen peroxide, and the breakdown of polyunsaturated fats.*

NAC and Glutathione

N-acetyl-cysteine (NAC) is a compound in the body used to recycle glutathione in the liver. NAC is made from cysteine, which is found in high-protein foods. NAC supplements may be taken with liposomal glutathione or as an affordable alternative, especially in the case where liposomal glutathione has been taken already or glutathione levels are good. (SpectraCell Laboratories offers testing for glutathione levels.) NAC, like glutathione, has numerous anti-inflammatory benefits, especially ones for the brain, liver, and thyroid.

What to expect if you choose to supplement? Given all the benefits above, people typically feel pretty good on a glutathione supplement. If you have not done much body cleansing or natural detoxification from the standard American style of eating beforehand, you may experience some signs of detoxification with the first few doses. Typically, any type of reaction improves very quickly (within a week or less), especially if the food plan is good and other support for proper digestion and detoxification are in place.

Chapter 5: Preparing for Your Cleanse

Planning will be vital for the success of any cleanse. Without proper planning, a cleanse will be cumbersome and tedious to follow. However, if you have all the ingredients, food items, and fluids at home, it will be much easier. Set aside time in your schedule to be well prepared.

Food Sources

- **Local farmers' markets and community-supported agriculture shares (CSAs):** Farmers' markets are a great source for seasonal vegetables and meats. Food from your local farmers' market or a CSA share is generally better than food from the store. The fresher the better!
- **Health food stores:** Shop for high-quality, locally grown meats and produce and fermented vegetables.
- **Organic:** Purchase organic fats, vegetables, and proteins. At a minimum buy organic for protein and Dirty Dozen foods (see www.ewg.org).

Cooking Equipment & Gadgets

- **Cookware** like stainless steel, cast iron, CorningWare, ceramic, and glass are superior and non-contaminating. Phase out aluminum and Teflon cookware, as they add heavy metals and toxins to the food.
- **Good chef's knife.**
- **Wood or bamboo cutting board.**
- **A salad spinner** to dry your greens for salads.
- **Glass containers** to pack your food.
- **A lemon juicer** to make juicing lemons more efficient.
- **A spiralizer** for cutting veggies into shapes like chips or noodles.

Water

Consider purchasing a filter for your water source if you do not already have one. A basic carbon filter will work as a start. Spring or alkalized water is best for drinking for most people, and it is important to eliminate the extra chlorine added to municipal drinking water.

Eating Practices

Before you begin a meal, focus on tuning in to your body and your emotions associated with food and sensations in your body.

Eat until you are 80 percent full, leaving 20 percent room for digestion. The metaphor of a washing machine can be helpful when it comes to your digestive system. Just like clothes do not benefit from an overstuffed washer, your digestive system needs room to do its work most efficiently and thoroughly.

Hunger is a common symptom in cleansing, especially if you are overcoming sugar addictions (cane sugar, flour products, chocolate). To help yourself, eat more fat and protein, and eat snacks more regularly. Eat mineral-rich foods, such as green drinks, sea salt, and lemon water.

Raw foods are very cleansing, so if you want a deeper cleanse and have strong digestion, you may want to emphasize them during the cleanse. If you have weak digestion, tend to get cold easily, or are doing this at a time of year when you feel cold, then cooked foods may be better for you. Similarly, juicing raw vegetables offers an opportunity for deep cleansing. This is okay so long as you are not too cold and have strong digestion. Be careful of too much sugar in the juice from sources such as beets and carrots. Light steaming, roasting, or stewing methods typically provide the easiest form of vegetables to digest.

Supplements

These supplements are recommended to support you throughout the cleanse (more info in Appendix C):

- Body Tune-Up Liver Support
- Liposomal glutathione (for more, see Chapter 7's section "Glutathione: An Amazing Antioxidant")
- Digestive enzymes
- Multivitamin
- Green drinks

To make long lasing effects, the meals and routines you establish in the Body Tune-Up must become habit. A woman undertook the Body Tune-Up due to chronic pain from migraines that affected her daily. She worked a demanding job that required her to put in ten to twelve hours daily. Prescription medications had been unsuccessful in managing her pain, and she sought the cleanses because a friend had told her about them. After two weeks on the cleanse, she began to experience a reduction in pain. The process of making time for herself and having total control over the food she ate eliminated most of her pain. She would shop and organize her meals on the weekends so she had food during the week. At my suggestion, she also took a turmeric supplement and vitamin D as indicated in her blood work to help improve her body's resilience and reduce inflammation. She continued to live pain free for about two years after the workshop ended. The last I heard from her, she was still working overtime, had stopped preparing her own meals, and was experiencing chronic pain again.

Exercise

Continue to get daily exercise, but do not overdo it. Listen to your body's cues; rest when your body is tired so that your energy can be used for cleansing.

Bowel Movements & Avoiding Constipation

You can expect to have some interesting bowel movements and urination (more and different types, colors, and sizes of elimination than usual) as your body is cleansing and shifting to a new food plan. When cleansing, be sure to drink plenty of water. Drink half your body weight in ounces of water every day. If, when coming into the cleanse, you do not have at least one easy bowel movement daily, start taking a magnesium supplement daily to remedy this. Additional suggestions for helping with elimination are discussed in the Digestive Cleanse section.

Body Care & Household Cleaners

A food-based cleanse is the perfect time to reassess the products you use on your skin and in your home, as they may contain toxins.

Skin Products

A good rule of thumb is to not apply anything you would not eat. Read the labels! Coconut oil, jojoba oil, olive oil, almond oil, and aloe vera are wonderful for your skin.

Cleaning Products

Products you use to clean your house can be toxic to the lungs and skin. They place added stress on your liver and other organs and glands. Look for products (dish soap, detergent, cleaning solutions, etc.) that say nontoxic.

In addition, a water filter on your shower helps reduce added chlorine.

Epsom Salts & Magnesium Baths

Magnesium sulfate is the scientific name for Epsom salts, which looks like table salt but is not for eating. Epsom salt baths are popular for relaxation, drawing impurities out of skin and relieving muscle aches, migraines, arthritis, and cold or flu symptoms. The magnesium and sulfates in Epsom salts are easily absorbed through the skin and may increase the magnesium levels in your body. This would be a great addition to the cleanse to pull extra toxins out of your body and help with possible symptoms of detoxing. Plus it will help you relax so you can sleep well while your body detoxes naturally.

Start with a quarter or half cup of Epsom salts in your warm bath, and soak for at least twenty minutes. Work your way up to two or three cups. A cup of baking soda may also be added, as well as magnesium chloride salts (one to three cups per bath), for additional benefits. Make sure to drink extra water during and after taking a bath to replenish liquids lost from sweating out the toxins. Taking this bath twice weekly is suggested.

Dry Skin Brushing: A Simple Tool for Health & Beauty

Your skin plays an important role in the process of eliminating toxins. Dry skin brushing is a simple and quick way to exfoliate and help the body detoxify naturally. It helps support the waste that may clog pores and helps you achieve a vibrant complexion. Dry skin brushing boosts the immune system, increases circulation throughout the body, and supports a healthy nervous system. Dry brushing carries nutrients to cells and stimulates the flow of the lymph, which will move the waste out. It also helps relieve organ congestion.

Always use a brush with natural fibers. A brush made with Tampico fibers from the agave plant is very effective. Use a softer brush on your face and neck. To achieve optimal results, body brush daily for a few minutes each time.

How to dry skin brush:

1. Dry brush your skin before you shower or bathe.
2. Start at your feet and brush toward your heart using long, even strokes.
3. Brush all the way up your legs, then over the buttocks, back, and abdomen. Concentrate on any areas that have cellulite.

4. Be sure to brush lightly on sensitive areas, like the breasts.

5. When you reach your arms, begin at your fingers and brush up your arms toward your heart.

6. Brush your shoulders and chest down, always toward your heart.

7. Avoid brushing anywhere the skin is broken or where you have a rash, infection, cut, or wound.

Alternating Hot & Cold Showers

Something as simple as taking a daily shower with alternating hot and cold water is reviving and supports healthy lymph. The lymphatic system is a network of vessels in our bodies that move the lymph, or extracellular fluid. This fluid helps move waste away from cells and plays a big role in the immune system too. Unlike the bloodstream, the lymph does not have a pump. When you are looking for an easy activity that results in healthy detoxification, immune system support, and improved circulation, alternating hot and cold showers fits the bill by stimulating blood and lymphatic flow.

Alternating hot and cold showers may be particularly helpful in cases of swollen lymph nodes, for example. It can also provide relief in cases of unexplained itching, which is sometimes a sign of stagnant lymph or a need for more detoxification support. Because the hot and cold showers promote expansion and contraction of the lymphatic system and blood vessels, circulation and cleansing are improved overall.

The hot water is stimulating and allows blood vessels to expand. Hot water helps move blood to the surface of the body. It is also relaxing and can help with headaches, including migraines, and muscle cramps.

Cold water is also stimulating but causes blood to move in the opposite direction, back to the core of the body and its internal organs. It causes the blood vessels to contract initially. After a period of time under cold water, the blood vessels expand again. Cold water encourages increased oxygenation and carbon dioxide excretion throughout the body. Cold water has been shown to increase metabolic activity of cells, boost antioxidant production, and both red and white blood cell formation. Overall, cold water therapy is invigorating.

This technique has merit as a lifelong practice and is also beneficial during the Body Tune-Up to help encourage rejuvenation.

How to take an alternating hot and cold shower:

1. Begin your shower as you typically would, with hot water.

2. After at least three minutes in the hot water, turn the dial to cold.

3. You may want to start with cold water on your feet, then hips, then shoulders, and finally your core and your head. Stay under the cold shower for at least thirty seconds.

4. Alternate back to hot and cold for thirty seconds each as many times as you wish, but end with a cold shower.

Additional Supportive Activities

- Deep-breathing exercises
- Increased sleep
- Near-infrared light/sauna

Chapter 6: Proper Food Combining

The purpose of following the food combining principles during the cleanse is so that you may digest foods better. This section is to help answer questions that may arise about selecting foods during the cleanse and to provide you with information about how each food group is digested.

The main proper food combining principles to observe are:

1. Eat fruit alone. Do not combine fruit, such as berries or apples, with proteins, fats, or vegetables. Lemon juice is the exception to this, as it can aid digestion.

2. Do not combine starchy foods (like grains or winter squash) with protein (like fish, eggs, or beef).

Vegetables *(consult the food combining list for each specific cleanse)*

Nonstarch or mild-starch vegetables (which would exclude things like potatoes and corn) take about five hours to digest, but they do not require strong acidic or alkalizing conditions in the digestive tract, so they combine with just about everything (except fruit!).

Fats

Fats are essential for helping your body deal with the toxins you release. They help your cells open up and release toxins. Fats require bile, an alkaline secretion from your liver and gallbladder, and lipase, an alkaline enzyme, to digest. Fats take about twelve hours to digest and, taken in small quantities, can be digested with all other food groups. Choose cold-pressed organic fats. Eat at least two tablespoons per meal.

Avocado is a fat generally only recommended for those who feel they need a heavier food during the Digestive Cleanse. It is a very versatile food and combines well with starches, fats, and fruits, as well as vegetables. It is a high-histamine food and not appropriate in high quantities for people with histamine-related issues, such as allergies, rosacea, and chronic postnasal drip.

Beverages

Beverages are best taken away from meals so that you do not water down your digestive secretions, making them less effective. Wait one hour after a decent meal before consuming liquids. Small amounts of liquid (four to six ounces) are okay with meals, especially if you have not gotten all your water in for the day. Listen to your body regarding thirst.

Proteins

Proteins require an acidic environment to digest. They are best eaten with low-starch vegetables. Other acidic foods can help (e.g., lemons, tomatoes, vinegars). Protein is a good choice to stabilize the glandular system, including blood sugar. This is especially important if you are irritable when you need to eat or feel weak and light headed when you do not eat enough. Proteins should not be combined with starches (high-starch vegetables, grains, or fruits) during a cleanse.

Fruits

Fruit is discouraged on the cleanse. If you are eating berries or other low-sugar fruits, then eat fruits alone and on an empty stomach. Fruits take thirty minutes to two hours in digestion time, passing through the digestive system very quickly. If eaten with other foods (like starch or protein) that take three to five times as long, as the fruit is held up and starts to "overdigest," it creates unhealthy fermentation and promotes bad bacteria. This leads to poor assimilation of nutrients and may contribute to the environment for dysbiosis, where the gut bacteria are out of balance.

The Importance of Fats and Proteins in the Food Plan

This section presents information regarding the therapeutic benefits of animal meats, including:

- *Why eating wild and free-range animal products has greater health and environmental benefits than eating grain-fed animal foods*

- *Why lower levels of fiber may be helpful*

- *How more fat and fewer carbs improve health*

- *What is understood about ancestors from the archaeological record who ate a meat-based food plan versus a grain-based food plan*

Benefits of Protein

One of the beneficial qualities of animal meats, including fish, seafood, poultry, and red meats, is the high protein content. The word *protein* comes from the Greek *proteios*, meaning "first place" or "primary." Indeed, protein is a basic building block for many vital substances within the body. It is required for hormone production, for example. That means protein is critical for healthy moods and sexuality. A balanced response to stress relies on hormones and neurotransmitters that are constructed with protein. Additional benefits of protein include:

- helping build the immune system, the bones and muscles, and the cardiovascular system.

- producing healthy hair, skin, and nails.

- serving as backup fuel when carbs and fats are lacking.

- carrying oxygen in our blood cells.

- making up our chromosomes, which carry the genetic material we pass down to our children.

- repairing the body.

- being a part of the enzymes that are needed for digestion, elimination, and various chemical reactions.

- leveling out blood sugar issues, thereby reducing fatigue and cravings.

- replacing carbohydrate-rich foods in meals, thereby reducing inflammation stemming from excess insulin production and excess triglycerides and oxidized LDL cholesterol in response to the carbohydrates.

- providing raw materials for hormones, therefore supporting thyroid, adrenals, sexual health, and hormone balance.

- supporting a strong immune system to fight infections.

- reducing brain fog.

Most women need to digest a bare minimum of sixty grams of protein daily, often more if they are more active or under stress. Men often need even more. An online protein calculator can help with individualizing your daily protein requirements. The individual level of protein needed can be fine-tuned with nutritional laboratory tests and a knowledge of functional medicine ranges.

Animal proteins have a more complete amino-acid profile than plant protein, so it is easier to get protein needs met with animal foods in most cases. Animal flesh includes the nine essential amino acids needed to fulfill protein requirements. While plant proteins like rice and beans may be combined to total the nine amino acids needed, the plant proteins have various trade-offs that often aggravate someone with health issues.

Some trade-offs of plant proteins include:

- Grains and legumes are carbohydrate rich, leading to greater insulin production, which leads to more inflammation.

- Grains and legumes are typically high in lectins, plant-made toxins that can cause aggravation in the digestive system and bloodstream.

- Plant-based foods are often high in phytic acid, which can leach valuable minerals like calcium and magnesium from the body, thereby weakening bones and teeth.

To get the benefits from eating fish, poultry, or meat, one must digest it. Some people complain that meat feels like a brick in their stomach or that they experience constipation or bloating. This is a typical sign of low stomach-acid production, as are heartburn and acid reflux. Even if a person does not digest protein well, their body still needs it and likely needs it more than ever to get healthy! It is important to assess the need for stomach-acid support, which may be done quantitatively with simple laboratory testing by a knowledgeable health practitioner. Protein requires adequate stomach acid to activate the enzymes needed for digestion.

There are many remedies that help stimulate stomach acid, including raw sea salt, apple cider vinegar (add one tablespoon to six to eight ounces of water) and betaine hydrochloride. If you are taking prescription medications, you should check to make sure they are not contraindicated, as some medications thin the stomach lining. Taking one or two capsules with a meal typically helps with protein digestion. Additional dosing or different products are sometimes appropriate in individual cases, however.

Carbohydrates tend to suppress stomach-acid production for some individuals, so practicing proper food combining or following a ketogenic food plan (low carb) or carnivore food plan (zero carb) are some options for helping with digestion of protein also.

Stomach-acid production is important not only for protein digestion but also for minerals. Animal products are particularly high in many minerals, including iron, zinc, potassium, magnesium, calcium, sodium, phosphorous, and selenium. Individuals with suboptimal levels of these minerals often need stomach-acid support and find that eating animal products can be therapeutic.

Another therapeutic quality of animal food is the iron content. Foods contain two types of iron: heme and nonheme. Both are present in animal foods, but plant foods only contain the nonheme type, which is more difficult to absorb on average. Therefore, when working to optimize one's iron levels, it is often more therapeutic to prioritize animal sources of iron over plant-based sources. I often suggest red meat daily for someone with suboptimal iron levels. Low iron levels often also signify low digestive secretions and leaky gut, so these areas should be evaluated as well.

Benefits of Fats

The other major nutritional component of meats is the fat. Obviously, natural meats range in their fat content. Poultry tends to have the least amount of fat and greater levels of omega-6. Some fish, like sardines and salmon, and red-meat cuts can be much higher in fat than poultry and superior due to their high omega-3 fatty acid content. Fat, especially animal fat, is critical to health not only as a fuel but due to the vitamins it contains. The fat-soluble vitamins in animal foods include A, D, E, and K_2. Some people cannot convert the vegetable source provitamin A to vitamin A and need a supplement or more animal foods (like liver) to get adequate A.

Fats are critical for nervous system health, including the brain. The brain prefers to run on ketones (which come from burning fat) versus carbohydrates. Fat helps to repair and heal the tissues in the body. Fat as a fuel also produces less free radicals and is a "cleaner" fuel for the body than carbs. Fats are critical for hormone health, stress response, and fertility because the hormones required are made from combining a protein with cholesterol, which is supported by fat in the food plan.

Some people report problems digesting fat or say they do not feel well on a fat-based food plan. Much of this trouble can be resolved with proper support for the liver and gallbladder. Supplements and herbs that help with fat digestion include phosphatidylcholine, ox bile, beetroot powder, and bitter herbs, like burdock and dandelion root. The Body Tune-Up Liver Cleanse formula is designed to help with fat digestion and is safe for most to take daily for maintenance.

Free-Range and Pastured vs. Conventionally Raised Animals

Free-range and pastured animals will provide more dense nutrition in terms of fat-soluble vitamins. The same is true for other nutrients in the fat from free-range animals, including beneficial omega-3 fatty acids.

Animals that are pastured or grass fed tend to be higher in omega-3 content and lower in omega-6. This is because animals that eat grass and other wild organisms are typically higher in omega-3 fatty acids naturally. Animals fed a grain-based omega-6-heavy food plan will end up with higher levels of omega-6 in their flesh. Choosing animal foods with a higher omega-3 level is generally better for Americans who tend to get too much omega-6 versus omega-3. An ideal ratio of omega-6 to omega-3 is about four to one. Choosing pastured and grass-fed animal foods and especially wild seafood helps balance this ratio by increasing the omega-3s. Individual omega-6 and omega-3 ratios may be measured with lab work. Those individuals with higher omega-6 levels tend to have more issues with high cholesterol levels and inflammation.

A common sign of omega-6 dominance (meaning your omega-6/omega-3 ratio is too high) is hives or other signs of high histamine levels (e.g., chronic allergies and rashes). Another common sign is dependence on ibuprofen, aspirin, or acetaminophen for relief from symptoms. These over-the-counter pain relievers work on reducing pain along the omega-6 pathway and are a typical sign that more omega-3s are needed and that there are too many omega-6-based foods in the food plan. Omega-6s are provided by vegetable oils and grains (canola, soy, sesame, safflower, sunflower, corn, avocados, etc. and their oils). Omega-3s are provided by fish and seafood and free-range animals that eat natural foods instead of grains. When you are shopping, look for pastured pork, for example. Look for eggs and chickens that are soy free, as some studies indicate typical chicken may have an omega-6/omega-3 ratio of thirteen to one, compared to soy-free chickens, which had an ideal ratio of four to one.[1] Beef should be 100 percent grass fed as well. It tends to be higher in omega-3 (from eating grasses) as well as some key amino acids and vitamins.

Animal meats have other benefits over plant-based foods in some cases. Plants contain lectins, which are toxins the plant uses to defend itself in nature. For people with aggravated or stressed immune systems and leaky gut, the high-lectin plant foods can continue to aggravate the problem. This has led many people to follow special low-lectin food plans promoted by authors like Steven Gundry avoid those plants highest in lectins. Many have found success on a carnivore food plan where they eat meat and fat only from animals to the exclusion of plant foods. For many, this approach can be very helpful and sustainable.

Unfortunately, many Americans still minimize animal foods for fear that they will increase their risk of heart disease. For many, this is not helpful for health. It appears that substituting vegetable oils for saturated fats potentially may increase the risk of death and that carbohydrates (yes, even the whole grains and especially gluten) contribute to a greater risk developing chronic disease than animal foods. This seems to be in part because carbohydrates contribute to high triglyceride levels, small dense LDL cholesterol, and advanced glycation end products (or AGEs), which are believed to contribute to disease.

Couch Potato Test

When we eat carbohydrates, the liver often makes triglycerides to store them. Have you ever eaten a big carbohydrate meal (like a plate of pancakes) and needed to lie down on the couch afterward? That is what it typically feels like to make triglycerides. It takes a lot of energy, and the body is taking the carbohydrates you just ate and storing them as fat. Some people experience this sleepiness issue after meals simply from eating a salad. This is often a sign of rising insulin and blood sugar difficulties and can be remedied through a change in food plan and supplementation.

A low amount of fat in the food plan will typically relate to lower HDL numbers, which further puts a person at higher risk for heart disease. One of the best studies we have to date indicates that the highest risk for coronary disease comes from a high triglyceride/low HDL ratio. Once we recognize these new understandings, it appears that reducing carbohydrates and increasing healthy saturated and unsaturated fats (rather than the other way around) help us to be healthier. Indeed, this is what I and many other health professionals see in consulting practice.

Furthermore, there are many new studies, including meta-analyses, that demonstrate that high-fat, low-carbohydrate food plans are more effective in reversing obesity, diabetes, and dementia than the low-fat standard food plans do. It is time to take another look at grass-fed and free-range or wild meats and their fats and consider the health benefits.

What about the lack of fiber?

Some critics of animal foods in the food plan may claim that the lack of fiber contributes to health issues. However, it appears that conventional wisdom around fiber may be another item that we did not know as much about as we thought we did. Many people suffering from constipation, for example, are concerned that meat does not contain enough fiber. However, to date, there has not been a peer-reviewed randomized and controlled study demonstrating that fiber benefits those with constipation. The only quality study that looked at fiber and constipation showed that those who reduced dietary fiber saw a reduction in their constipation. Those who eliminated fiber completely from the food plan saw an elimination of negative digestive symptoms.

What do records of ancient people tell us about their eating habits and health?

Evaluating the evidence of what paleolithic or ancient people ate and their health status can help us with understanding optimal food choices. Experts claim that our genetics and the related physiology we have today were developed throughout the past. Michael Eades, retired MD and health blogger, states that 99.6 percent of all generations of Homo species had no experience with modern foods. Therefore, if we want to understand what foods may work best for us, it is helpful to study ancient peoples and what they ate.

We will never know 100 percent what ancestors ate; however, scientists have used evidence to compare meat-eating hunter-gatherers to farmers, whose food plan relied on grain. They found that the ancient meat eaters had much healthier teeth and bones, reflecting superior nutritional status. For more information on this, see Dr. Eades's video *Paleopathology and the Origins of the Paleo Diet*. He explains that the Egyptians' so-called "healthy" food plan, which relied heavily on wheat, vegetables, and fruits, with sparse amounts of red meats, likely contributed to the very high rates of heart disease detected from soft-tissue samples of ancient Egyptians.

Weston A. Price, a Canadian dentist, also studied ancient food plans. He presented information resulting from his international survey of aboriginal peoples eating traditional food. He recorded the healthiest populations based on teeth and jaw health and concluded that the most robust individuals relied heavily on animal foods.

Ethical and Environmental Considerations

Although there are many nutritional benefits to eating animal foods, critics argue that a vegetarian food plan is healthier for the environment and more ethical to animals. Author Lierre Keith takes this on in her book *The Vegetarian Myth*, where she argues that a heavy reliance on plant-based foods, like grains and legumes, produced in an agricultural setting equates to biologic cleansing and habitat destruction. The loss of wild habitat, soil, and diversity caused by farming alone is important to consider when making an ethical choice about food planning.

Factory farming of animals is a horrendous practice and should be stopped. However, free-range grazing of animals can be done in an ethical manner. Furthermore, regenerative agriculture demonstrates that grazing animals can restore biological diversity in the soil and native habitats. Grazing of animals in natural habitats like prairie can help with slowing or reversing global warming through carbon sequestration. Keith encourages us to consider that we can make better food choices through supporting sustainable agriculture that includes animal husbandry.

Summary

Animal meats contain beneficial nutrients, including protein and fat, vitamins, and minerals. There are many reasons why an animal-based food may be therapeutic. Choosing animals that are free range, wild, or pastured and soy free is critical.

Part 2: The Cleanses — Doing the Work

Chapter 7: Digestive Cleanse

10 DAYS

When your body is eliminating toxins, those toxins pass through the colon, or large intestine, before they leave. If your colon is blocked or not fully functioning, the toxins and metabolic wastes you are cleaning from your cells will be reabsorbed. This will work against your efforts at cleansing. A healthy colon will typically have two to three bowel movements daily if you eat two to three major meals.

Besides its role in digestion and elimination, the gut also plays a role in mental health. The majority of serotonin and dopamine, important neurotransmitters for mental health, are made in the gut. Approximately 15 percent of the intestinal lining is composed of enteric endocrine cells, which produce over 90 percent of the serotonin and over 50 percent of the dopamine neurotransmitters. The brain does not produce most of its own neurotransmitters; the gut does! Because of this, the Digestive Cleanse will often provide improvements in cognitive and emotional wellness as well.

In addition to improving the functioning of the colon and gut lining in this cleanse, we also need to improve the level and diversity of good bacteria in the gut. You can do this by taking a product called ION* Biome, probiotics, and/or fermented foods (unless you have histamine issues) and eating well.

Using proper food combining and avoiding inflammatory foods, the Digestive Cleanse is a great start for many suffering from acid reflux. It allows digestive secretions to normalize and helps reduce the inflammation contributing to the symptoms. For example a middle-aged woman came to me with a bad case of acid reflux. It would make it difficult for her to sleep at night and would often occur at any time of the day, even with just drinking water. She received permission from her doctor to try making dietary changes instead of taking a prescription medication for a short period of time. She went through both the Digestive and the Critter Cleanses and then moved on to a maintenance food plan with my direction. Within the first few days, she experienced a drop in the severity and occurrence of acid reflux. Several years later, she is still free from this problem by continuing to eat well.

The purpose of the Digestive Cleanse is to:

- help cleanse and eliminate debris from your digestive tract.
- provide awareness regarding your digestive habits (such as chewing, time of food in digestive tract, and bowel regularity).
- establish a regular habit and taste for healthy foods (and possibly discover new dishes that you love to cook!).
- balance your metabolism and blood sugar levels.
- break your attachment to unhealthy foods.
- change the bacteria in your gut for the better.
- lay the groundwork for the next cleanses.

The protocol includes a food program of cleansing foods. Supplements are taken to bind undigested debris and toxins in the colon and add healthier bacteria.

Major cleansing concepts we are working with include:

- eating lightly to give your body extra energy to do internal "housekeeping" by giving it a break from all the work to process the more inflammatory foods and complex meal combinations.
- following proper food combining for better digestion.
- avoiding foods that are typical allergens and contribute to inflammation (wheat, corn, potatoes, sugar, chocolate, dairy, peanuts, and soy, for example).
- eating more nutrient-rich foods to support multiple body systems.
- feeding beneficial bacteria a healthy food plan to improve digestion, immune health, detoxification, and mental health.

I suggest you begin a journal of your experience. It can be as simple as a few notes next to Day 1, Day 5, and Day 10. Or it could be a detailed meal-by-meal diary to help you zero in on the foods that are causing you issues. If you have time, keep track of your foods, activities, emotions, physical sensations, and so on. This can be a resource for you as you introduce foods later or do a food-based cleanse in the future.

What to Expect

You may experience:

- more frequent hunger.

- more bowel movements than normal. Alternatively, you may experience constipation (see "Regular Bowel Movements—Very Important!" later in this chapter).

- feeling lighter and more focused.

In order to curb negative side effects, follow these suggestions:

- Eat more often if you are hungry, especially more fat like olive oil. Always have a healthy snack on hand, such as a cup of broth or soup or chopped vegetables. Plan ahead!

- Eat the recommended vegetables and fats for breakfast, snacks, lunch, and supper.

- Take a few tablespoons of healthy fats each day (in homemade salad dressings or added to vegetable juice is okay), such as olive oil or cold-pressed flax oil. These are anti-inflammatory and help improve detoxification.

Food Recommendations

- Do not eat after 8 p.m.
- Chew food thoroughly.
- Drink plenty of water (half your body weight in ounces of water daily). This can come by way of herbal teas, fresh vegetable juices (only low-carb; avoid carrot juice, for example), and green drinks.
- If you find you do not feel satisfied with meals, add in one or two palm-size servings of lean protein at each meal. This will help you feel fuller and stabilize blood sugar. The protein will provide multiple benefits.
- Avoid very cold food, especially if you tend to feel cold. Let raw food warm up on the countertop before you eat it or use it in a smoothie, for example. Heat food if it is still cold.

Fats

- **Yes:** First cold-pressed olive oil, flaxseed oil (in salad only or at medium-low heat), hempseed oil (salad only), unrefined coconut oil (good for high-heat cooking). Unrefined is very important for all these oils. Lard, duck fat, and other natural animal fats are also beneficial for cooking at high heat.

- **No:** Butter; margarine or other processed oils; store-bought salad dressings or spreads; refined or expeller-pressed oils; clarified butter (ghee).

Vegetables

- **Yes:** Raw, frozen, steamed, baked, sautéed, juiced, or boiled vegetables. Especially dark leafy green vegetables (try to eat at least one per day of kale, chard, collards, turnip greens, beet greens, dandelion greens, etc.). Green drink. Note that members of the tomato family/ nightshade vegetables (tomatoes, peppers, eggplant, potatoes) tend to encourage inflammation for some and should be reduced or avoided.

The nightshade family also includes cayenne pepper, chili powder, and paprika.

- **No:** Canned vegetables. Corn or potatoes in any form. Avoid nightshade vegetables (tomatoes, peppers, eggplant, chili peppers) if you have inflammation issues (stiffness or pain).

Proteins

- **Yes:** Organic and free-range or wild sources only (includes fish, bison, elk, beef, turkey, venison). Eggs should be from cage-free, soy-free chickens. (Note: Eggs are a common allergen, so you may want to avoid them in the cleanse). A collagen powder like Great Lakes gelatin. Spirulina and chlorella are also sources of protein and may be purchased in powders and added to water or in pill form.

- **No:** Conventional meats or vegetarian meat products. No soy.

Soups

- **Yes:** Homemade soups made from allowed ingredients. Use the leftover water from steaming or boiling vegetables as a stock. See Supportive Recipes section for suggestions. Homemade stocks from organic animal meat or bones are good.

- **No:** Store-made stocks containing nightshade vegetables (potatoes, tomatoes, bell peppers, eggplant, hot peppers, tomatillos, paprika, pimentos), natural flavors, or sugars. Bouillon cubes or packaged mixes. Canned or packaged soups.

Salad Dressings & Toppings

- **Yes:** Homemade dressings (see Dressing and Sauce Recipes section).

- **No:** Mayonnaise, bacon bits, croutons, any prepared dressings (read labels) that include refined oils, soy, dairy, sugar, natural and artificial emulsifiers, coloring, preservatives, et cetera.

Starch, Grain, Legumes, Nuts, & Seeds

- **None.** It is not advised to eat a lot of starchy, high-lectin foods such as these during cleanses because they can trigger inflammation and intestinal permeability (leaky gut) for many people, especially those with autoimmunity diseases and weakened immune systems. For some people with food sensitivities, even flaxseed may not be advisable.

Dairy

- **None.** (Not even butter, cheese, kefir, clarified butter, or yogurt!)

Condiments

- **Yes:** Sea salt, organic herbs and spices, mustards made with apple cider vinegar, kimchi, fresh sauerkraut.

- **No:** Soy sauce; tamari sauce; prepared ketchups and mustards; refined and filtered vinegars; any condiments containing sugar, corn syrup, sorbitol, et cetera. Coconut aminos are okay sparingly.

Spices

- **Yes:** Herbs and natural spices including but not limited to basil, chives, cilantro, cumin, curry powder, garlic, oregano, parsley, sea salt, sea veggies, thyme, turmeric, et cetera.

- **No:** Spice mixes that include table salt ("salt"), sugar, or anything artificial. Avoid cornstarch and other corn derivatives, like dextrose.

Beverages

- **Yes:** Half your weight in ounces of water daily. Distilled or filtered water is best. Have at room temp or warmer. Herbal teas are acceptable. Fresh vegetable juices. Homemade broths (no potatoes).

- **No:** Coffee, soda, caffeinated beverages, milks (of any kind), cocoa, sweetened juices, or beverages containing "natural" or "artificial" flavorings, preservatives, or sugars.

Sweeteners

- **Yes:** Licorice root pieces or powder (this is different from the candy), but not if you have high blood pressure tendencies. Carrots, beets, and berries, while not technically sweeteners, can help a sweet tooth.

- **No:** Stevia, pure maple syrup, raw honey, blackstrap molasses, brown rice syrup, agave nectar, corn syrup, sucrose, white sugar, brown sugar, dehydrated cane sugar, turbinado sugar, sorbitol, NutraSweet, Sweet'N Low, saccharin, or other artificial sweeteners.

Fruits

- **Yes:** Fruits are high in sugar and should be eaten minimally, no more than one serving daily, if at all. Fruits eaten should be raw, baked, poached, or frozen, organic, and very low in sugar. Avoid any fruits you are sensitive or allergic to. Berries or tart apples are best because of the lower sugar content and high amount of vitamin C.

- **No:** Bananas or other tropical fruit, fruit drinks/juices, prepared lemonades or bottled teas, dried fruit.

Dessert

- If you have sweet cravings, you should eat more protein and fat to better nourish your body. You may also try to add in more sweet veggies, like carrots and beets, and a little extra fruit, but this may make it harder to get into ketosis or burn fat.

- **No:** Sweetened or prepared desserts, ice cream, candy, chocolate (no cocoa in any ingredient list).

Proper Food Combining Chart

How to read this chart: Foods that may be combined at a meal are connected by a line.

Starches and fruits should be taken minimally.

PROTEINS
Beef, Bison, Cold-Water Fish, Turkey

NONSTARCHY VEGETABLES
Arugula, Asparagus, Bamboo Shoots,
Beet Greens, Bok Choy, Broccoli,
Brussels Sprouts, Cabbage, Cauliflower,
Celeriac, Celery, Collard Greens,
Cucumbers, Endive, Fennel, Garlic,
Green Beans, Jerusalem Artichokes,
Jicama, Kale, Kohlrabi, Leeks, Microalgae,
Mushrooms, Onions, Peas, Radishes,
Seaweed, Shallots, Sprouts, Summer
Squash, Swiss Chard, Zucchini

STARCHES
Carrots (minimal)

FRUIT
Berries (minimal),
Cranberries, Lemons,
Limes

FATS & OILS
Cold-Pressed Oils (Coconut, Flax,
Olive), Duck Fat, Lard

SPECIAL FOODS
Apple Cider Vinegar, Bone Broth,
Cultured Vegetables, Sauerkraut

Supplements

Supplements are often used with a cleanse to accelerate the effects. The bentonite "shake" or G.I. Detox capsules described here are an optional component of the Digestive Cleanse that act as a binder to help pull out toxins and extra debris from the digestive system. You may continue longer with one of them if you like the results, as they are safe for long-term use.

Bentonite shake

With plenty of water, take this bentonite drink away from meals. The shake may be taken on an empty stomach in the afternoon, instead of before bed. Combine the ingredients below. Shake up and drink quickly.

How to make the shake:

- 1 Tbsp liquid bentonite, Sonne's #7 Detoxificant (or ½ tsp dried bentonite, though it is chalkier)
- 1–2 Tbsp ground flaxseed or other ground fiber (gluten free, like psyllium husk) or Ortho Molecular Products' Fiber Plus Powder. *Note: If you have a sensitive digestive system or many food sensitivities, you may be sensitive to the flaxseed or psyllium (it is a high-lectin food, and some high-fiber foods feed a microbial overgrowth). In that case, you may want to omit the ground flaxseed/fiber for several days to notice any effects.*
- 8 oz water

G.I. Detox capsules

G.I. Detox, produced by Bio-Botanical Research Inc., is a pill alternative to the bentonite shake, acting as a binder to help remove toxins. Take two G.I. Detox before bed on an empty stomach with plenty of water.

Healthy gut bacteria supplements

To add healthy bacteria to the digestive tract and provide you with enough energy while cleansing, take the following daily with meals or away from meals:

- **Cultured vegetables:** 1–2 Tbsp (kimchi or live sauerkraut) with meals to provide probiotics. Watch for added sugar. Avoid if you have issues with yeast/candida or have histamine issues.
- **Probiotics:** Take one capsule of Body Tune-Up Multistrain Probiotic daily on an empty stomach or with meals.
- **Digestive enzyme:** To support weak digestion, you can take Allegany Nutrition's digestive enzymes. Betaine and Pepsin are helpful if protein causes gas and bloating.
- **Green drinks:** Drink one or two daily. Examples of green drinks can be found in the Drink Recipe section.

Regular Bowel Movements—Very Important!

If you are not passing two easy bowel movements a day, support the body by trying one or more of these strategies:

- *Add more fat (e.g., olive oil, fish oil).*
- *Add more sea salt (e.g., add two teaspoons to two cups of hot water and drink first thing in the morning).*
- *Take four tablespoons ground flax daily or a soft fiber supplement.*
- *Take one or two tablespoons of black sesame seeds daily.*
- *Drink plenty of fluids (water, broths and herbal teas). Have a green drink daily.*
- *Add gentle, non-habit-forming herbal supplements, such as Triphala or Super Aloe capsules.*
- *Improve your stomach-acid production and bile flow with digestive enzymes and probiotic supplements. Liver Lover tea and the Body Tune-Up Liver Cleanse supplement also may help.*
- *Eat stewed prunes (one or two at a time) if you are not avoiding fruits.*
- *Add a magnesium supplement, like Mg-Zyme, in the evenings for constipation. Increase the dosage until the constipation is resolved. Many adults may need 600 mg or more per dose.*
- *Gargle multiple times daily to stimulate the vagus nerve.*
- *Consider colon hydrotherapy and enemas.*

Daily Protocol

For meal ideas, take a look at the twelve-day menu plan in the Recipes section, or build your meal plan based on the Food Combining Chart.

Upon waking
Optional: Body Tune-Up Multistrain Probiotic and 4 oz water.

Advanced: *Self-care time—do some journaling, meditation, deep breathing, gratitude list, et cetera*

Pre-Breakfast (15 minutes before eating)
Optional: 1 tsp of ION* Biome

Breakfast
Choose a suggested meal from the menu, or create a meal of your choice per the plan.

Midmorning snack
Ideas include:
  • Fresh veggies
  • Green drink
  • Broth—bone or vegetable
  • Herbal tea

Pre-Lunch (15 minutes before eating)
Optional: 1 tsp of ION* Biome

Lunch
Choose a suggested meal from the menu, or create a meal of your choice per the plan.

Afternoon snack
Ideas include:

- Chopped veggies with homemade dressing or dip
- Leftover soup
- Kale crunch
- Green drink
- Herbal tea

Pre-Dinner (15 minutes before eating)
Optional: 1 tsp ION* Biome

Dinner

- If you have not had one yet, sip on green drink or herbal tea (ginger or peppermint, for example) while cooking dinner.

- Choose a suggested meal from the menu, or create a meal of your choice per the plan.

"Dessert"
Chamomile or other herbal tea, green drink, et cetera.

Don't eat after 8 p.m.

Bedtime
Bentonite with fiber/flaxseed shake, or 2 capsules G.I. Detox (optional).
This may be moved to the morning if desired.

Beverages
See Drink Recipes section for beverage ideas.

The Leaky Gut and Inflammation Connection

Over 70 percent of the total immune system cells are in the gut. If there is dysfunction in the gut, there is dysfunction in the immune system. Conversely, if there is an immune system issue, suspect a gut permeability issue. Because the immune system reaches all areas of the body, the immune activity in the gut has an effect throughout the entire body.

When activated too often, these gut immune cells trigger the release of proinflammatory chemicals. Just like it sounds, such chemicals promote inflammation. During acute stress, the pain and inflammation in a healthy individual are quickly resolved by anti-inflammatory compounds. However, when the gut is under stress all the time in a common condition known as leaky gut syndrome, or hyperpermeable intestines, the immune response promoting inflammation can go on much longer and become chronic.

Leaky gut means the tight junctions in the gut lining have become "lax" and the integrity of the digestive tract as a filter is reduced. Foods and viruses, for example, that should not get into the body's bloodstream may enter and the immune system becomes more activated, resulting in chronic inflammation and autoimmune activity. The name "leaky gut" sounds gross, but in fact, experts believe most people experience it at some point in their lifetime. Leaky gut syndrome can manifest in many different ways that may seem unrelated to digestion at first glance. Frequent illness (viral and bacterial infections), autoimmune conditions, blood sugar disorders, allergies, skin problems, gastrointestinal disorders, joint pain, nervous system and mood disorders, and even coronary heart disease all may be attributed to leaky gut.

Experts believe that leaky gut is a precursor to the development of autoimmune activity. Leaky gut develops when the level of a key antioxidant, glutathione, is depleted. Glutathione depletion occurs through aging, poor food choices, exposure to toxins, and chronic stress. (For more on glutathione, see Chapter 4's section "Glutathione: An Amazing Antioxidant"). Once leaky gut develops, the antibody-secreting immune cells flag undigested protein segments from food that enters the bloodstream. They can also flag our own tissues. Some foods trigger stronger antibody production and pro-inflammatory chemical release than others. Gluten, dairy, and soy are examples of such foods. Eliminating these common allergens leads to a reduction in chronic pain and inflammation. This is a major reason why these foods are not eaten during the cleanses.

Experts also think that the levels of lectins or toxic compounds in a food correlate with the level of inflammation perpetuated by the food. This may be another reason why "elimination periods" low in cereal grains and high in vegetables, natural fats, and wild or free-range animal-based proteins appear to relieve chronic inflammation when followed for an extended period of time (at least several weeks). Processed sugars, or too much sugar, also perpetuates pro-inflammatory chemical release through the presence of insulin. Therefore, any approach toward dietary improvement needs to include sugar reduction.

A Tour of the Digestive Tract

Do you know when digestion first begins? You might respond "When you chew," but the digestive process begins in your brain upon thinking about that meal you are going to eat. The hypothalamus, which is a gland at the base of brain, begins to send signals to the salivary glands in the mouth and other parts of the digestive tract to prepare the body for the meal.

Cleanse Tip! Once you are sitting down to eat, obviously chewing the food is essential, and it is often lacking. The yogis say you should chew once for every tooth you have. If you do this, you will find your food is a paste before you swallow. This is a good exercise to do if you are seeking better health and digestion. Only by chewing the food into a paste and coating it in salivary enzymes do you optimize the beginning of the digestive process. To enhance digestion in this segment of the cleanse, set your fork down between bites, and chew the food until it is a paste before swallowing.

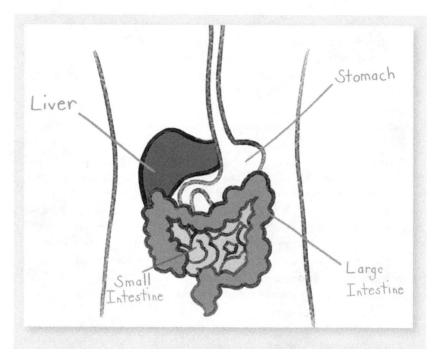

Enzymes, organic molecules that act like a key unlocking the molecules of food so they can be better broken down and absorbed, are released by salivary glands in the mouth. There are many types of enzymes, ranging from ones that break down starches (amylases) and ones that break down fats (lipases) to ones that break down proteins (proteases). When we chew food and coat it in saliva, these enzymes go to work. This mixture is then swallowed and enters the esophagus.

The food, coated with enzymes and saliva, will ideally sit in the bottom of the esophagus and upper stomach for twenty to thirty minutes. During this time, the salivary enzymes are digesting the food and the stomach is creating an acid bath as the stomach expands to receive the meal. To enhance digestion at this phase, you may take a digestive enzyme supplement with your meal. This adds extra digestive enzymes to help enhance the breakdown of foods to nutrients.

The acid bath, composed of hydrochloric acid, potassium chloride, and sodium chloride, is critical for the digestion of proteins and minerals, as it activates pepsin. Without adequate acid bath in the stomach, absorption of proteins and minerals may be insufficient for optimal health. Acid also kills harmful bugs you might pick up from travel or from a bad salad bar. Most important to people who suffer from acid reflux: the acid signals the closing of the esophageal sphincter. Without this closing, the acid that is made will erupt from the stomach when it uses mechanical action for digestion. The stomach has strong muscles in its lining that help churn the food to support better digestion.

Many people with heartburn or acid reflux have insufficient stomach acid and, contrary to popular belief, will get relief from doing things to encourage more acid, like:

- Adding one tablespoon of apple cider vinegar to a small glass of water with a meal
- Taking a betaine hydrochloride supplement with meals to help increase more acid production, like Ortho Molecular's betaine and pepsin or Biotics Research Hydro-Zyme
- Increasing sea salt in their food plan, like Baja Gold sea salt

If the above items do not agree with the person, or they make the reflux worse, then this a sign there is likely too much inflammation occurring in the upper digestive tract for the proper acidic environment to be supported. The solution in this case is to reduce the inflammation in the stomach lining. A gut health formula including glutamine, zinc carnosine, and herbs may be helpful in resolving this stage. Once inflammation is reduced, then steps to encourage stomach-acid production may be resumed.

The stomach churns the food and bathes it in acid until it becomes a liquid we call "chyme." The chyme then is released at the bottom of the stomach into the small intestine. While this process is occurring, the body is taking inventory of the composition of the chyme: Is it fat? Protein? Whatever kind of enzymes needed to break down the chyme is then sent from the pancreas to the small intestine.

The pancreas makes a variety of enzymes to break down various nutrients and will send this "cocktail" to the gut, where the enzymes coat the chyme. Low pancreatic enzyme production may be a result of low stomach acid. The pancreas also releases sodium bicarbonate to the small intestine.

Simultaneously, bile is secreted from the liver and gallbladder through the bile duct to the small intestine. Bile helps break fats apart so that the lipase made in the pancreas can break fats down further to be absorbed across the intestinal lining. Bile also helps trigger the bowel movement so that any food waste lower down in the system continues to move out. One other thing about bile and sodium bicarbonate is their alkalinity (meaning they are high on the pH scale, the opposite of acid). Alkaline bile and bicarbonate mixing with acidic chyme (which is acidic because it just came from the stomach) creates a pop and sizzle not unlike those volcanoes at elementary science fairs where baking soda and vinegar are combined. This chemical environment allows for the further breakdown of food into basic nutrients that can be moved across the gut lining in the small intestine.

Many people's issues with digesting fat may be rooted back to the body not making or releasing bile when it is needed. Besides increasing sea salt (like Baja Gold) in the food plan, eating adequate fats, and supporting proper stomach-acid production, there are supplements like Body Tune-Up Liver Support by Human Nature that are very helpful with releasing bile for fat digestion.

When the gallbladder struggles to release the bile, a person may have gallbladder attacks, constipation, or diarrhea. While most people choose surgery to remove the gallbladder, there are natural remedies and changes in food plan that can help avoid surgery for some. I come from a line of women with gallbladder attacks and have experienced them myself, and I have found natural supplements and food plan changes to bring relief and resolution of this issue.

The gut lining is only one cell layer thick. This allows for the easy transfer of nutrients into the bloodstream below. In this way, the digestive system is like a filter, only allowing nutrients across, while indigestible things and bad bugs we might be exposed to continue to move through the colon to be excreted. Many people experience "leaky gut" or hyperpermeable intestines, which sets the stage for food sensitivities, infections, autoimmunity issues, and disease to develop. One of my favorite supplements that helps leaky gut is ION* Biome by Biomic Sciences.

The gut biome comprises the bacteria and other microbes that reside throughout the entire digestive tract. The mouth has different species of bacteria than the esophagus, which is very different from the acid-tolerant bacteria in the stomach, for example. The bacteria throughout the gut help with the breakdown and absorption of food and the production of stool to be excreted as a bowel movement from the colon. Due to the use of antibiotics, poor-quality food, and other stressors, it can be very helpful to take a probiotic supplement to help recover digestive health. Prebiotics, which are food for the beneficial bacteria, may be found in foods like garlic, onions, chicory, and many others.

Nutrients and water from the food continue to be absorbed as the stool is moved from the small intestine through the colon and finally excreted through the anus. When regular bowel movements, such as two or three per day, do not occur, then the waste from this process can present a stress to the body, as it may become overburdened by waste materials that are designed to be moved out but instead become reabsorbed into the bloodstream. The key to addressing bowel regularity lies in supporting the steps of digestion already discussed and often changing the food plan. Natural laxatives may remedy the problem but may be habit forming and cause problems with prolonged use. One approach that often helps constipation is to time meals so that there is at least a three-to-four-hour break between them.

Those with loose stools and diarrhea may also need assistance with proper digestive secretions. However, they also typically require a shift in food plan and lifestyle to promote a healthier gut biome and reduced inflammation.

Histamine Intolerance

Many individuals have signs of histamine intolerance and benefit from avoiding high-histamine foods. Symptoms of histamine intolerance often mimic allergy symptoms and may include rash, hives, headache, rosacea, diarrhea, postnasal drip, runny nose, itchy eyes, low blood pressure, asthma, sinus symptoms, flushing, and slow or irregular heart rate.

A histamine intolerance develops when too many histamines accumulate in a body and exceed the body's ability to break them down. Histamine is typically broken down in the gut, so signs of histamine intolerance can often point to leaky gut. Therapies that help identify the root cause of leaky gut and then help repair and heal the gut lining can be instrumental in overcoming a histamine intolerance. The bacteria in the gut also generate histamine, and some species of bacteria generate more histamine than others. Therefore, a histamine intolerance may also be a sign that the bacterial balance in the gut is off, a condition called "gut dysbiosis." In this case, stool testing that identifies the root cause of a gut imbalance is valuable in rehabilitating the gut and overcoming histamine intolerance. The Digestive Cleanse and Critter Cleanse in the Body Tune-Up are helpful strategies for improving gut health in these areas as well. Histamines are also affected by hormones whereby estrogen dominance leads to higher histamines.

While working to address the root cause of a histamine intolerance, it can be helpful to follow a low-histamine food plan. Histamine is formed as a breakdown product in perishable food, in microbial fermentation and maturation processes, and in the ripening of fruit. Even some vegetables naturally contain histamine, although very fresh. Histamines are highest in:

- Fermented or microbially ripened products (for example, alcoholic products, vinegar, yeast, and bacteria)
- Perishable fresh produce with inadequate/uncertain freshness
- Canned or processed foods
- Kept warm or reheated food (especially fish, meat, and mushroom dishes)

Avoid these high-histamine foods:

- *Fish, if not freshly caught or frozen*
- *Meat, if no longer fresh, such as sausages and dry-cured meats*
- *Aged cheese, processed cheese (histamine increases with aging)*
- *Any fermented food, like sauerkraut and kimchi*
- *Tomatoes, spinach, eggplant, avocado*
- *Alcoholic drinks, fermented fruit juices, kombucha*
- *Vinegar, pickled vegetables*
- *Soy sauce, Worcestershire sauce*

The foods and additives listed below can release endogenous histamine from certain cell types in the body (mainly from mast cells). This mechanism is independent from poor breakdown of histamines discussed above and can happen in a healthy person if they consume excess:

- *Alcohol (ethanol)*
- *Strawberries*
- *Nuts (walnut, cashews)*
- *Seafood, shellfish, crustaceans*
- *Chocolate, cocoa*
- *Tomatoes, ketchup, tomato juice*
- *Citrus fruits*

Often a supplement that works as a natural antihistamine can help provide relief from symptoms in an individual with histamine intolerance. I suggest a blend of quercetin, NAC, and nettles or butterbur in a supplement. See Appendix C.

Chapter 8: Critter Cleanse

14 DAYS

The purpose of this Critter Cleanse is to help balance your intestinal ecosystem. The protocol includes a food program for strengthening and nourishing your body with wholesome foods. You have been eliminating the foods that feed overgrowths of bacteria, yeast, and other critters like worms in the previous Digestive Cleanse. This is helpful, as many unhealthy symptoms are derived from an imbalance in the gut biome. We will now add natural supplements to help eradicate unhelpful critters and encourage the growth of beneficial ones.

The importance of addressing gut dysbiosis is supported by numerous scientific studies that demonstrate a connection between an imbalance in the gut biome, or overgrowth of certain species, and health problems.

During the Critter Cleanse, you will use the Body Tune-Up Critter Cleanse supplement, a blend of antimicrobial and antiparasitic herbs, to potentially reduce organisms that can get established in the gut and contribute to health issues. Different organisms such as bacteria, yeast, and protozoa, when in an overgrowth state, reduce digestive secretions such as stomach acid and pancreatic enzymes. This further contributes to malabsorption, nutrient deficiencies, digestive issues, and histamine overload. The Critter Cleanse described here is a shortened version, just fourteen days, of what I would typically suggest to someone when we do a comprehensive stool test (I prefer the GI-MAP test by Diagnostic Solutions) and identify dysbiosis and unwanted organisms. Therefore, if you find you benefit from the two weeks on the critter herbs, or you have an interesting experience, you may want to consider taking them longer or working with a practitioner that can guide you further.

The justification for doing the Critter Cleanse prior to the Kidney and Liver Cleanse is that the latter cleanses will be more effective and go more smoothly if the gut environment is in tip-top shape and well supported. The herbs included in the Critter Cleanse not only act as natural antiparasitics but also boost digestive secretions and are high in antioxidants.

Some people are understandably resistant to doing a Critter Cleanse without any evidence of a problem. You may refer to the chart in the Appendix that lists common symptoms of gut dysbiosis as a reference. A GI-MAP stool test is an excellent way to determine if the Critter Cleanse is necessary, if there is doubt. Furthermore, I can attest to hearing positive feedback about the Critter Cleanse over the years from people who were initially unsure about it.

A woman did the Body Tune-Up because she wanted to learn more about natural foods and eating well. She and her husband had been unable to conceive and as a result had adopted children. She was initially resistant to the Critter Cleanse because she lived with her husband, kids, and dog and felt it might be pointless. I encouraged her to go through with it anyway. Several weeks later, she managed to do the cleanse and shared with me she was so glad she did because she passed several globs of mucus and other interesting things in her stool while taking the Critter Cleanse herbs. Fast-forward a couple years, and I received an update from her that she was pregnant. She felt that the path she started with the Body Tune-Up toward eating better overall had led to the improvement in health that allowed her to conceive and deliver a healthy child.

What to Expect

You may or may not experience the following:

- **Unusual cravings and dreams.** These may be caused by die-off from the Cleanse. Do not indulge in strong cravings for sugars, processed carbs, and unhealthy foods. Try water with sea salt, lemon, and apple cider vinegar, a high-dose probiotic, or a green drink to help reduce cravings. Eat more protein and fat for satiety.

- **Feeling tired.** As the critters die off, the elimination organs of the body may be overwhelmed, leading to a feeling of fatigue. If this happens, back off a bit and slow down the cleansing by reducing your activities or reducing the dosage of the supplements temporarily. Drink plenty of fluids, and try the bentonite shake again. G.I. Detox capsules also help with this.

- **Interesting bowel movements.** It is good to keep tabs on the condition of your bowel movements so you can know if anything interesting happens! It is common for people to become constipated when eradicating parasites, and a fiber supplement and herbal support like Ayur-Triphala will help with elimination. G.I. Detox also helps with this. *For additional tips on maintaining regular bowel movements (at least two per day), see the "Regular Bowel Movements—Very Important!" chart in Chapter 7.*

- **Abdominal pain.** It is uncommon, but some people experience abdominal pain (like gas) if they are expelling a critter. Drink plenty of chamomile tea and receive colon hydrotherapy as needed.

Food Recommendations

Continue eating the same foods as you were during the Digestive Cleanse. For the Critter Cleanse, you may add/emphasize these foods:

Fats

You may add avocado, coconut, and coconut milk (unprocessed). These are a combination of protein and fat. Please note these may be high in histamines, so be careful if you tend to have high-histamine issues.

Spices

Consider incorporating spices with antiparasitic properties, such as fennel, clove, cayenne (avoid if you are not eating nightshades), sage, ginger, oregano, horseradish, and thyme.

Starch

You may add these starchy vegetables, but avoid them if you want to stay ketogenic: acorn squash, beets, butternut squash, delicata squash, pumpkin, winter squash, parsnips, rutabaga, and spaghetti squash.

Nuts & Seeds

You may add pumpkin seeds, if desired, unless you have autoimmune tendencies, in which case introduce these carefully, if at all. (Nuts and seeds are sometimes difficult to tolerate in autoimmune cases.)

Additional Suggestions

- At each meal, add in one palm-size serving of protein, such as fish, beef, turkey, or bison, if you desire, and have not been doing this since the first cleanse. This will help you feel fuller and stabilize blood sugar. Spirulina and chlorella are also good sources of protein and may be purchased in powders and added to water or smoothies.

- Eat plenty of garlic, cabbage, leeks, onion, radish, kelp, and raw sauerkraut. Beets are also antiparasitic (but are not ketone promoting).

- Try eating a small handful of raw or roasted pumpkin seeds daily as an additional antiparasitic protocol.

- Avoid overeating. Eat until 80 percent full. End your meal with high-fiber food to help digestion.

- Chew food thoroughly.

Proper Food Combining Chart

In the chart below, foods that may be combined at a meal are connected by a line. Foods in **bold** are new for this cleanse phase.

Fruits should be taken minimally. Starches listed may be combined with other foods at meals (but not if ketogenic).

PROTEINS
Beef, Bison, Cold-Water Fish, Turkey

NONSTARCHY VEGETABLES
Arugula, Asparagus, Bamboo Shoots, Beet Greens, Bok Choy, Broccoli, Brussels Sprouts, Cabbage, Cauliflower, Celeriac, Celery, Collard Greens, Cucumber, Endive, Fennel, Garlic, Green Beans, Jerusalem Artichokes, Jicama, Kale, Kohlrabi, Leeks, Microalgae, Mushrooms, Onions, Peas, Radishes, Seaweed, Shallots, Sprouts, Summer Squash, Swiss Chard, Zucchini

STARCHES
Acorn Squash, Beets, Butternut Squash, Carrots, **Delicata Squash, Parsnips, Pumpkin, Rutabaga, Spaghetti Squash, Turnips, Winter Squash**

FATS & OILS
Avocado, Coconut (unsweetened), Coconut Milk, Cold-Pressed Oils (**Borage,** Coconut, **Fish,** Flax, **Grapeseed,** Olive, **Sesame**), Duck Fat, Lard, **Pumpkin Seeds**

FRUIT
Berries (minimal), Cranberries, Lemons, Limes

SPECIAL FOODS
Apple Cider Vinegar, Bone Broth, Cultured Vegetables, Sauerkraut

Supplements

The Critter Cleanse requires herbs taken every day for fourteen days or longer. Also, be sure to restore good bacteria with the daily Body Tune-Up Multistrain Probiotic and/or fermented vegetables (if you do not have histamine issues).

Protocol

Take the Body Tune-Up Critter Cleanse capsules fifteen to thirty **minutes prior to each meal (three times per day).**

Days 1–14: Take two capsules three times daily before meals.

—OR—

If you are very sensitive to herbs when you begin, cut back your amount accordingly and increase by one capsule every day until you are at the full dose of two capsules before three meals daily.

For Maintenance

Two capsules three times per day before meals, once a week.

Daily Protocol

The following protocol is the same as the Digestive Cleanse, with the addition of the Body Tune-Up Critter Cleanse supplements.

For meal ideas, take a look at the twelve-day menu plan in the Recipes section, or build your meal plan based on the Food Combining Chart.

Upon waking
Optional: 1 capsule Body Tune-Up Multistrain Probiotic and 4 oz water.

Advanced: *Self-care time—do some journaling, meditation, deep breathing, gratitude list, et cetera*

Pre-Breakfast (15 minutes before eating)
- 2 capsules Body Tune-Up Critter Cleanse
- *Optional: 1 tsp ION* Biome*

Breakfast
- Meal of your choice (based on Food Combining Chart)
- Try to eat within 30 minutes of waking to stabilize blood sugar.

Midmorning snack
- Ideas include:
  - Fresh veggies
  - Green drink
  - Broth—bone or vegetable
  - Herbal tea

Pre-Lunch (15 minutes before eating)
- 2 capsules Body Tune-Up Critter Cleanse
- *Optional: 1 tsp ION* Biome*

Lunch

- Meal of your choice (based on Food Combining Chart)

Afternoon snack

- Ideas include:
  - Chopped veggies with homemade dressing or dip
  - Leftover soup
  - Kale crunch
  - Green drink
  - Herbal tea

Pre-Dinner (15 minutes before eating)

- 2 capsules Body Tune-Up Critter Cleanse
- *Optional: 1 tsp ION* Biome*

Dinner

- If you have not had one yet, sip on green drink or herbal tea (ginger or peppermint, for example) while cooking dinner.
- Meal of your choice (based on Food Combining Chart)

"Dessert"

Chamomile or other herbal tea, green drink, et cetera

Don't eat after 8 p.m.

Bedtime

Bentonite with fiber/flaxseed shake, or 2 G.I. Detox capsules

Beverages

See Drink Recipes section for beverage ideas.

Chapter 9: Kidney Cleanse

4 DAYS

The purpose of the Kidney Cleanse is to support the kidneys in the elimination of metabolic waste that builds up in the bloodstream and kidneys. This four-day protocol will also help reduce the level of detrimental acids, like uric acid, that go into the bloodstream. The protocol includes a food program of cleansing foods. Herbal supplements in the Body Tune-Up Kidney Support capsules are taken to support the kidneys and bladder based in part on the work of Hulda Clark. The kidney drink and capsules also support the liver and gallbladder and help prepare you for the Liver Cleanse.

What to Expect

New practice:

- **Slow, all-day sipping.** You will have to gradually sip the kidney drink throughout the day. Keep your focus on the cleanse so that you do not forget to sip.

You may experience:

- **a lag in energy.** This may be most prominent during Days 1 and 2. **Do not overtax yourself,** or you may become sick. Keep activity to a lower level, and rest as needed. Avoid strenuous exercise. Any out-of-the-ordinary exercise that is not a part of your daily routine may overtax your body, and your cleanse will not be productive.

- **more frequent urination.** The herbal remedies are natural diuretics, so drink plenty of water and eat plenty of vegetables.

- **possible unusual bowel movements.**

- **aches or soreness in the middle back.** The kidneys work hard to eliminate debris. If you notice pain in your middle back, plan to cut back on the amount of kidney tea you are taking by half, and get plenty of rest. Drink plenty of warm water. Eat foods high in vitamin C. Consider enemas and colon hydrotherapy if you become too uncomfortable.

- **minor physical discomforts.** Your body is catching up with the detoxification and adjusting to the herbs.

Food Recommendations

Continue eating the following foods as you were during the Critter Cleanse. For the Kidney Cleanse, you may add/emphasize these foods:

Fruits

You may add cherries for their benefit to the kidneys (avoid too many if ketogenic).

Nuts & Seeds

You may add flax seeds, chia seeds, and almonds (avoid too many if ketogenic).

Legumes

You may add white or cannellini beans if you are not satisfied at meals without the animal protein and generally appreciate eating beans. Soak and prepare your own beans (see Supportive Recipes section). If you have issues with intestinal permeability, then you may want to avoid or be extra cautious with adding legumes. (Legumes are not on a ketogenic food plan.)

Additional Tips

- Continue to eat many vegetables with healthy fats, keeping meals simple. If you do not have much of an appetite, eat lightly.
- Drink plenty of water (half your body weight in ounces daily). Lemon water, ginger tea, or warm water are good.
- Do not drink more than one cup a day of additional herbal tea (such as nettle or chamomile tea) during the four-day Kidney Cleanse to keep diuretics under control.
- Avoid excessive salt, including sea salt, during the four days.
- Traditionally kidney cleanses have not included animal proteins. If you need protein, choose fish, turkey, or other protein easy to digest.
- Take a break from other supplements. Kidneys filter all that goes in your body, so supplements and medications create extra work.

Proper Food Combining Chart

In the chart below, foods that may be combined at a meal are connected by a line. Foods in **bold** are new for this cleanse phase. Fruits should be taken minimally. Starches listed may be combined with other foods at meals (but not if ketogenic).

PROTEINS
Beef, Bison, Cold-Water Fish, Turkey, **White Beans**

NONSTARCHY VEGETABLES
Arugula, Asparagus, Bamboo Shoots, Beet Greens, Bok Choy, Broccoli, Brussels Sprouts, Cabbage, Cauliflower, Celeriac, Celery, Collard Greens, Cucumber, Endive, Fennel, Garlic, Green Beans, Jerusalem Artichokes, Jicama, Kale, Kohlrabi, Leeks, Microalgae, Mushrooms, Onions, Peas, Radishes, Seaweed, Shallot, Sprouts, Summer Squash, Swiss Chard, Zucchini

STARCHES
Acorn Squash, Beets, Butternut Squash, Carrots, Delicata Squash, Parsnips, Pumpkin, Rutabaga, Spaghetti Squash, Turnips, Winter Squash

FATS & OILS
Avocado, **Almonds, Chia Seeds,** Coconut (unsweetened), Coconut Milk, Cold-Pressed Oils (Borage, Coconut, Fish, Flax, Grapeseed, Olive, Sesame), Duck Fat, **Flax Seeds,** Lard, Pumpkin Seeds

FRUIT
Berries (minimal), Cranberries, Lemons, Limes

SPECIAL FOODS
Apple Cider Vinegar, Bone Broth, Cultured Vegetables, Sauerkraut

Supplements

The four-day Kidney Cleanse requires a homemade herbal tea mixed with parsley broth and flavored with optional black cherry extract. It also requires supplements to be taken each day. Make the Kidney Drink the day before you begin the cleanse, if possible.

Kidney Drink Ingredients

- **¾ cup Kidney Cleanse Tea** (hydrangea root, gravel root, and marshmallow root). Open the box and measure this out per the "Decoction" recipe below. This tea is composed of hydrangea, which is a natural diuretic, meaning that it increases the filtering function of the kidneys. This may cause increased urination. The gravel root is designed to help soften metabolic waste, such as kidney stones, that becomes compacted in the kidneys, so that it may pass out of the body without issue. The marshmallow root is anti-inflammatory and soothes and balances the effect of the other two herbs. If you are taking a medication that has a diuretic mechanism, you should check with your doctor before adding in the Kidney Cleanse Tea, which has a diuretic action.

- **1 bunch fresh parsley.** Parsley is a natural diuretic that supports increased kidney function.

- **Black/Tart cherry concentrate.** The cherry concentrate includes dark antioxidants known as anthocyanins that have been shown reduce the levels of uric acid in the bloodstream. Excess uric acid is known to cause issues with memory and, in extreme cases, a condition called gout. If you are sensitive to sugar and enjoy a ketogenic food plan, then you may want to leave the cherry concentrate out of the Kidney Cleanse, as the cherries have it has natural sugars.

Equipment

- Large nonmetal container, such as a glass bowl, jar, or pot with a cover
- Cooking pot (may be metal)
- Nonmetal strainer (cheesecloth, bamboo strainer)
- 2–3 sterile pint- or quart-size jars with lids
- Freezer containers for leftovers

Kidney Cleanse Tea Decoction Preparation

1. Brew the tea by filling the nonmetal container with 10 cups of filtered water. Add the ¾ cup of roots and mix into water. Cover. Soak for 4 hours or overnight. (If you wish, you may cut the water and herbs in half to make less.)

2. Pour roots and soak-water into a cooking pot and bring to a boil. Turn heat down and simmer for 20 minutes, covered.

3. Strain into a nonmetal container, then pour into a sterile pint jar and keep in the refrigerator. Makes 10 cups, so the remaining tea should be stored in freezer containers to be used in subsequent Kidney Cleanses.

4. To resterilize, bring to a boil. *The soaked roots can be saved and used one more time, so freeze them too. Boil the presoaked frozen roots in 10 cups water for 10 minutes to make the tea.*

Parsley Broth

1. Rinse the fresh parsley. Bring one quart of filtered water to a boil.

2. Drop parsley in water and boil for 3 minutes. Strain and pour into sterile pint jar. Keep in the refrigerator. Makes 4 cups. (You will only need 1 cup or less, so freeze the rest or use it as a soup base.) The boiled parsley can be added to a soup or vegetable sauté, or you can discard it.

Begin the Cleanse

The Kidney Drink

Each morning for Days 1 and 2, combine in a mug:

- ¾ cup Kidney Cleanse Tea decoction
- ½ cup parsley broth
- 2 Tbsp black cherry concentrate

The Kidney Drink is your "special drink." You do not have to heat the drink, but you may. **Drink it evenly over the day; do not drink this all at once or you will get a stomachache and feel pressure on your bladder.**

On Days 3 and 4, you may stop the drink, but continue to take 2 Tbsp black cherry concentrate daily in warm water or a smoothie.

Body Tune-Up Kidney Support Capsules

During each of the four days of the cleanse, take two Body Tune-Up Kidney Support capsules two times daily with meals. The vitamin B_6 and magnesium in the formula have been shown in clinical studies to reduce the development of kidney stones and support healthy kidney function. The resveratrol is a superfood that is high antioxidant and anti-inflammatory. The Chinese salvia extract in the capsule improves kidney activities.

Summary Calendar of Four-Day Cleanse

Item	Day 1	Day 2	Day 3	Day 4	Maintenance
Kidney Drink	Yes	Yes	*Stop	*Stop	Stop
Black Cherry in water	(included in Kidney Drink)	(included in Kidney Drink)	Yes (~2 Tbsp) with water	Yes (~2 Tbsp) with water	Continue if you wish, but use 1 Tbsp or less daily
Body Tune-Up Kidney Support capsules	Yes	Yes	Yes	Yes	Continue if you wish until gone

*The original protocol for the cleanse is to do the tea each day for four days. You may do this if you wish to have a deeper cleanse. Back pain and/or low energy while on the Kidney Cleanse are indicators that two days of tea are enough for you. It is better to cleanse less if you are unsure than to overcleanse on this one.

Daily Protocol

For meal ideas, take a look at the Recipes section, or build your meal plan based on the Food Combining Chart.

Upon waking
Optional: 1 Body Tune-Up Multistrain Probiotic capsule and 4 oz water

Advanced: *Self-care time—do some journaling, meditation, deep breathing, gratitude list, et cetera*

Pre-Breakfast (15 minutes before eating)
- *Optional: 1 tsp ION* Biome*
- Begin sipping Kidney Drink, and sip all day long

Breakfast
- Take 2 Body Tune-Up Kidney Support capsules
- Meal of your choice (based on Food Combining Chart)

Midmorning snack
- Ideas:
  - Pumpkin seeds
  - Veggies with a dip from the Dressing and Sauce Recipes section
  - Green drink

Pre-Lunch (15 minutes before eating)
- *Optional: 1 tsp ION* Biome*

Lunch
- Meal of your choice (based on Food Combining Chart)

Afternoon snack
- Ideas:
  - Chopped veggies
  - Soup
  - Green drink

Pre-Dinner (15 minutes before eating)
- *Optional: 1 tsp ION* Biome*

Dinner
- Take 2 Body Tune-Up Kidney Support capsules
- Meal of your choice (based on Food Combining Chart)

Bedtime
Bentonite with fiber/flaxseed shake, or 2 G.I. Detox capsules (optional)

Beverages
See Drink Recipes section for beverage ideas

Chapter 10: Liver Cleanse

12 DAYS

Until this point, the program for the Body Tune-Up has focused on supporting detoxification in the liver. The purpose of this twelve-day Liver Cleanse protocol is to support your liver and gallbladder with nutrition and allow these organs to move out stagnant bile or gallstones, thus supporting Phase 3, or the Elimination Phase, specifically. While not the focus, the liver does continue to experience the supporting effects of the other phases of detoxification.

You will avoid the foods that are harmful to the liver, take a tea or tablets for support, and follow a two-day apple fast and a liver-cleansing cocktail. The protocol here is adapted from the liver cleanse originally proposed by Hulda Clark.

The day after the liver-cleansing cocktail will be a day to rest as the toxins work their way from the liver to the gallbladder and out of your body via the bowel and kidneys, primarily.

What to Expect

- **Down time.** Take it easy on Days 11 and 12. Be prepared to fully rest on Day 13, the day after the liver-cleansing cocktail. Make sure your schedule allows for this.

- **Some physical discomfort.** Nausea or headaches may be experienced on Days 11–12 and the day after the cleanse. This happens as your liver catches up to the release of toxins. Ginger tea, capsules, and baths will help with the nausea, as will resting. White willow bark is a supplement that helps with headaches. A colonic or enema will enhance the results of the cleanse and provide relief if nausea is present.

- **Strong emotions.** A congested liver can be associated with strong emotions such as anger and irritation. Do not indulge in strong emotions as they arise. Write them down and let them go. Meditate and breathe deeply. Take a gentle walk or nap.

- **Unusual bowel movements after Day 12.** Look for small green pea-shaped bile secretions and gallstones.

- **Sugar cravings.** You may have strong sugar cravings after the Liver Cleanse if apples are too high in sugar for you. Resist sugar! Find enjoyment in things like carrots, Star's lemonade (see the Drinks Recipes section), fats, and monk fruit sweetener. Avoid very cold or frozen drinks, as they will be too stressful for your system initially. Eat proteins and fats that are easy to digest for satiety.

- **Additional urination.** The digestive tract, liver, and kidneys all work together to cleanse the body. It is not uncommon for a Liver Cleanse to manifest a strong elimination from the kidneys, for example, in the form of urination.

Food Recommendations

Days 1–10

Same foods as the Kidney Cleanse.

Days 11–12

These are the apple days. Eat an apple when you are hungry. If you are avoiding excess sugars, Granny Smith apples may be a good choice. You may also eat low-starch vegetables if you want to avoid apples altogether. Drink plenty of water. Do not eat fats. Do not take any supplements that are not completely necessary. If you cannot make it through two days of just apples, you can shorten this to one day and do the flush that first night. Or you may eat steamed veggies instead of apples, but no oil or other fats.

Day 13

This is a day of rest. Eat lightly when you are hungry.

Proper Food Combining Chart

Foods in this chart that may be combined at a meal are connected by a line. Fruits should be taken minimally. Starches listed may be combined with other foods at meals (but not if ketogenic).

PROTEINS

Beef, Bison, Cold-Water Fish, Turkey, White Beans

NONSTARCHY VEGETABLES

Arugula, Asparagus, Bamboo Shoots, Beet Greens, Bok Choy, Broccoli, Brussels Sprouts, Cabbage, Cauliflower, Celeriac, Celery, Collard Greens, Cucumber, Endive, Fennel, Garlic, Green Beans, Jerusalem Artichokes, Jicama, Kale, Kohlrabi, Leeks, Microalgae, Mushrooms, Onions, Peas, Radishes, Seaweed, Shallots, Sprouts, Summer Squash, Swiss Chard, Zucchini

STARCHES

Acorn Squash, Beets, Butternut Squash, Carrots, Delicata Squash, Parsnips, Pumpkin, Rutabaga, Spaghetti Squash, Turnips, Winter Squash

FRUIT

Berries (minimal), Cranberries, Lemons, Limes

FATS & OILS

Avocado, Almonds, Chia Seeds, Coconut (unsweetened), Coconut Milk, Cold-Pressed Oils (Borage, Coconut, Fish, Flax, Grapeseed, Olive, Sesame), Duck Fat, Flax Seeds, Lard, Pumpkin Seeds

SPECIAL FOODS

Apple Cider Vinegar, Bone Broth, Cultured Vegetables, Sauerkraut

Supplements

This twelve-day Liver Cleanse consists of a careful food plan for ten days and liver-supporting tablets. Days 11 and 12 consist of apple fasting, which ends with drinking an olive oil/lemon cocktail on the last night. On Day 13, be sure to rest and allow your body to eliminate thoroughly.

The intent of this protocol is to cleanse the liver and gallbladder of stagnant bile, the end products of Phase 1 and 2 detoxification, so that the liver will function in a more balanced manner. The Liver Support tablets help to prepare your body for the cleanse. The bitter-tasting tea and herbs stimulate specific taste buds at the back of the tongue. This signals the parasympathetic nervous system to trigger a number of reflexes. The stimulation of digestives juices promotes the flow of bile, which assists the liver in its detoxifying capacity. The apples, high in malic acid, pectin, and enzymes, soften thick bile and help to release bile when the olive oil/lemon cocktail is consumed.

Days 1–10

Take two tablets of Body Tune-Up Liver Support with at least each meal daily. It is good to chew the tablets for the best benefit.

If you are taking a prescription medication that acts as a diuretic, you should consult your doctor before taking the Liver Support tablets, because they also have a natural diuretic component.

Days 11 & 12 (apple days)

Start the mornings by eating an apple when you are hungry. Tart apples are best, but any apple you like is okay. Ideally you do not take any of your supplements these two days. Throughout the day, eat another apple as you become hungry. You may bake the apples (six apples will bake for 40 minutes at 375° in a covered dish; you can add a little lemon juice and cinnamon before baking).

It is okay to eat some vegetables if you need to. Do not eat fat, because we want to build up bile for these two days prior to the liver-cleansing cocktail. Do not eat after 7 p.m. Avoid laxatives and oils for these two days.

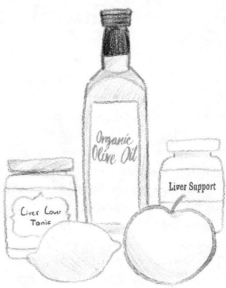

For a gentler cleanse: Fast on apples for one day instead of two, therefore taking the olive oil/lemon juice cocktail at bedtime on the eleventh day.

If eating only apples for two days will not work for you, you may take malic acid powder in water (or capsules) instead to get the same benefits. In this case, eat vegetables (but no fat) for the two days. Raw vegetables, cooked vegetables (steamed or boiled), and vegetable broth are acceptable alternatives to eating apples.

If taking malic acid, mix one teaspoon of powder with thirty-two ounces of water and divide into three parts to drink throughout the day. Rinse your mouth with water and baking soda afterward to protect your teeth from the acid. Drink plenty of water. If you choose malic acid capsules, take two capsules three times daily with or without vegetables.

The apples and malic acid help to soften the bile. Avoiding fat for two days helps with buildup of bile, so the release is greater on Day 13.

If you usually have trouble sleeping, drink peppermint, chamomile, passionflower, or skullcap tea in early evening. Use lavender essential oil or another calming blend in a diffuser or on your wrists.

Day 12 (night of the liver-cleansing cocktail)

- Stop eating at 5 p.m.

- Then, a half hour prior to bedtime (before 9:30 p.m. works best), pour three to four ounces 3–4 oz. of olive oil into a cup.

- Squeeze the lemons to make two to three ounces of juice, and combine with the olive oil.

- Mix by pouring from one cup to another twenty times, or use a pint jar with a cover and shake to mix.

- The flavors are strong, so drink quickly, and follow it by sucking on a wedge of lemon to cut any aftertaste.

Some find it easier to drink the olive oil if it is slightly warm (place the cup of olive oil into another cup that contains warm water), but others prefer to drink through a straw or have the olive oil chilled. Do what works for you.

The "old school" version of this cleanse includes a second olive oil/lemon juice cocktail thirty minutes after the first, so for a deeper cleanse, you may add this before you go to bed.

After drinking your cocktail, go to sleep (before 10 p.m. works best). Do not clean up the kitchen or do other chores; go to bed right away. If you think you may have a hard time sleeping, take some calming herbs, such as chamomile or ginger tea.

Doing colonics or enemas can help ease any discomfort or nausea you might experience, so these may be done in the days leading up to the cocktail or the days after.

Day 13 (next morning)

Plan to rest at home. Spend the time reading, relaxing, and meditating. Do a little bit of gentle exercise in the fresh air. Within twenty-four hours, you should expel stones, mucus, or sludge through bowel movements. Look for gallstones in the toilet with the bowel movement. There may be many colors, but the green ones, indicating bile, are common. **A colonic or enema** is recommended to help this process. A colonic before (Days 10–11) and after the cleanse (Day 13) is recommended.

If you are not hungry, then do not eat; simply drink water, tea, fresh diluted juice, et cetera. When you start eating foods again, be mindful about your choices: eat lightly and follow proper food combining principles. It is best to consume low-starch vegetables or green drink for the remainder of the day. If you are hungry, eat steamed veggies.

For some people, sugar cravings become stronger after a Liver Cleanse in association with the purge of yeast from the organs. Be mindful of this natural process, and avoid refined sugars and refined snack foods and flours afterward. You may take your parasite herbs afterward if you wish in a case like this.

If you don't feel satisfied with the results, you may repeat the flush in another two weeks. Never cleanse while ill. Never do this flush without doing the Critter and Kidney Cleanse first to prepare the body.

Sometimes the bile ducts are full of cholesterol crystals that did not form into round stones. They appear as "chaff" floating on top of the toilet bowl water. It may be tan colored, harboring millions of tiny white crystals. Cleaning out this chaff is just as important as purging stones.

Daily Protocol

The following daily protocol applies to Days 1–10. Days 11 and 12 are the apple days as described in the previous section.

For meal ideas, take a look in the Recipes section, or build your meal plan based on the Food Combining Chart.

Upon waking
Optional: 1 Body Tune-Up Multistrain Probiotic and 4 oz water

Advanced: *Self-care time—do some journaling, meditation, deep breathing, gratitude list, et cetera*

Supplements
- Chew or swallow whole 2 tablets Body Tune-Up Liver Support with each meal

Pre-Breakfast (15 minutes before)
- *Optional: 1 tsp ION* Biome*

Breakfast
- Meal of your choice

Midmorning snack
- Ideas:
  - Pumpkin seeds
  - Green drink
  - Broth

Note: If you have low energy, then vegetables would be a better snack at this time because they are not as cleansing

Pre-Lunch (15 minutes before)

• *Optional: 1 tsp ION* Biome*

Lunch

• Meal of your choice

Afternoon snack

• Ideas:
  • Chopped veggies
  • Soup
  • Green drink

Pre-Dinner (15 minutes before)

• *Optional: 1 tsp ION* Biome*

Dinner

• Meal of your choice

Bedtime

Bentonite with fiber/flaxseed shake or 2 capsules G.I. Detox (optional)

Beverages

See Drink Recipes section for beverage ideas

Chapter 11: After the Cleanse

You have done the hard work the previous six weeks and have eliminated the highly reactive foods and created a perfect situation for "testing" foods to which you may be sensitive. It is recommended that you maintain simple meals, slowly adding foods back in one at a time and observing their effects on your body.

When a food contains toxins or is not properly digested by your body, it may result in skin problems, inflammatory responses in the body, headaches, irritability, a change in energy or mood, et cetera. If you are a careful observer of the relationship of foods to your body, then you will be able to avoid unpleasant health issues in the future by adjusting your food choices to avoid the aggravating foods. A hypersensitivity to foods is a sign of leaky gut and will likely require natural supplements to overcome. We invite you to schedule a consultation with us if you would like support in this area.

Unfortunately, not all food sensitivities are obvious. There are some more insidious reactions to gluten and dairy, for example, that can lead to the destruction of brain tissue and the development of cognitive diseases like Alzheimer's. Blood sugar imbalances can similarly not always show up as symptoms yet may increase our tendency for issues later in life. Blood tests via Cyrex Labs can help identify existing immune reactions that may not otherwise be identifiable at this stage.

Sustainable Healthy Food Plan

This section is about how to choose foods for best vitality.

Food

- Every meal should consist of protein, fats, and nonstarchy vegetables. Some people may appreciate an additional half-cup serving or so of healthy vegetable starch, like sweet potatoes, beets, or plantains (but this amount of carbohydrates does not typically allow for ketosis and its benefits).

- Avoid falling into the habit of eating the same meals every day.

- Consume foods in moderation, and get a variety of them in type and color.

- Choose locally grown, organic foods as much as possible.

- Drink plenty of water (half your body weight in ounces daily for most people).

- Avoid overeating. Eat until 80 percent full, and end your meal with celery to help digestion.

- Chew food thoroughly.

- Do not eat after 7 or 8 p.m.

- Plan your meals, and prepare meals or ingredients ahead each week. Chop, slice, and precook ingredients for faster cooking time. Chop once, eat twice or more.

- Keep your refrigerator and pantry stocked with the staples you use each week.

- Snacks: Only snack when you are hungry, generally. Continue as you were. New snack ideas: organic beef jerky, hard-boiled eggs, roasted root veggies, seaweed snacks, or goat dairy.

- Eat processed foods and sugars very rarely, if at all.

- Life happens. You attend parties or eat out, and you can't eat every meal perfectly. Try to choose the best option on the table or menu, and don't feel guilty. If your regular daily meals reflect the foods you ate during the Body Tune-Up, then rare meals with other less-nourishing foods won't be a big deal. The ION* Biome and digestive enzymes can help reduce the impact of suboptimal foods on your gut health.

- When eating out, try to find restaurants that serve higher-quality foods, locally sourced ingredients, and farm to table. Avoid fast food.

Supplements

- Maintain a balance of vitamins, herbs, and minerals that give you a benefit. Each person's food plan has its deficiencies, so it can help with many issues to have routine blood work done at least once or twice yearly. At Human Nature, we offer a nonmedical evaluation of your chemistry to help inform what specific supplements may benefit you.

Maintenance Plan Post Tune-Up

Digestive System Maintenance Cleaning

- May take daily bentonite shake, G.I. Detox, and probiotics if desired.

Critter Infestation Prevention

- Body Tune-Up Critter Cleanse:

  - Take two capsules three times per day before meals daily for up to two to three months for difficult cases.

  - Two capsules three times daily before meals once a week may help with maintenance.

Kidney Support

- Add about a tablespoon or less of the tart/ black cherry concentrate to water, a smoothie, or other beverage daily.

- Green drinks, chlorella, or spirulina may be taken daily for support.

Liver Support

- Body Tune-Up Liver Support capsules may be chewed with meals for ongoing liver and fat digestion support.

Testing Period

Protocol

- As you add in new foods, try to space them at least one day apart so you can know if you have a reaction to something. Eat the new food times that day.

- Maintain the building blocks of the cleanse while adding in new foods. At each meal, eat protein, nonstarchy vegetables, and one to two tablespoons of added fat (like oils, nuts, seeds, avocado, etc.).

- If you have time, it's ideal to space new food introductions three to four days apart, as a food sensitivity might manifest over seventy-two hours in response.

- Common allergens that are most likely to cause reactions include gluten, sugar, dairy, eggs, citrus, corn, soy, white potatoes, and peanuts.

- Good foods to try first would be animal foods like pork, lamb, or chicken, as well as sweet potatoes, nuts, and seeds.

- Avoid fried foods, sugar, and flour products. You may want to avoid these foods for at least thirty days after the cleanse and even try to minimize them all the time for optimal health. Some people observe how great they feel without these foods and never add them back in.

- Be aware of high-histamine foods like avocados, citrus, chocolate, spinach, canned foods, and cured meats. If these and similar foods trigger a reaction, you may want to investigate a low-histamine food plan further and pursue additional work on your gut biome.

- Avoid foods you think you are sensitive to for at least another six weeks, and then you could try them again.

Support While Testing

- Fermented foods and probiotics, freshly squeezed vegetable juices, green drink, lemon drinks, multivitamin, liquid minerals, and digestive enzymes can be beneficial for the testing period and in the long term for maintaining health and energy levels. Vitamin D supplements or a vitamin D light may be valuable as well.

- Green drinks and foods like chlorophyll and spirulina will help your body to detox any bad food reactions.

- Occasional herbal blends and vitamins may help address specific nutritional needs.

- Homemade soups, broths, and vegetables will continue to be beneficial, as they were on the cleanse.

Other Ways to Test Foods

- **The Coca Pulse Test** is a simple technique involving taking your pulse before and after ingesting a food. See the book *The Pulse Test*, by Arthur F. Coca (1994).

- **Food sensitivity blood testing** is another way to gain information about your body's reactions to food. A blood test can determine antibody levels, which tell whether or not there is a strong immune reaction to a variety of foods. Testing is available through Human Nature. We suggest Cyrex Labs testing as the best in this field.

Chapter 12: Future Cleansing

After doing the Body Tune-Up once, you may want to repeat it, or just repeat sections of it. The information below provides some general guidelines for this.

- **Digestive Cleanse:** You may repeat as often as every six to eight weeks or quarterly. Remember that the Digestive Cleanse is the foundation for all other cleanses, so you may want to always do a Digestive Cleanse first for best results.

- **Critter Cleanse:** Someone who's more susceptible to parasites (for example, they work with animals or have a history of complex parasitic infections) would do the cleanse two or three times per year.

- **Kidney Cleanse:** You may repeat two to three times per year.

- **Liver Cleanse:** You may repeat as often as every eight weeks.

The entire cleansing series, including the elimination/testing period, may be repeated up to one to four times per year until most of your health issues are resolved.

If you would like to cleanse more frequently than is recommended, or you are unsure about how or when to cleanse, work with a professional to get more guidance.

Many who do the Tune-Up say that it helps them get a handle on otherwise uncontrollable cravings. It does this through eliminating common foods that trigger cravings and providing adequate nourishment to the body to help reduce the craving cycle. A middle-aged woman had struggled with overeating her entire life, especially with sugar. She had seen several alternative and functional health practitioners who had suggested diet change and supplements over the years. She would follow these programs for a while but then fall back into her old habits of compulsive eating. The Body Tune-Up proved to be valuable in providing a clear road map on how to eat better. I have known her for several years since her initial cleanse, and any time life takes her in a direction where she begins eating sugar again, she will use the food-based cleanses as an opportunity to reset. Her situation is not unique.

Part 3: Supportive Recipes

Digestive Cleanse Menu Plan

DAY	BREAKFAST	LUNCH	DINNER
1	• Option 1: Bowl of Soup or Broth (Bone or Veggie) • Option 2: Smoothie (Cleansing or Berry Green)	• Rainbow Salad • Lettuce Wrap with Meat of Choice	• Slow Cooker Ribs • Fried or Grilled Zucchini
2	• Bowl of Soup • Protein suggestions: Sardines, Ground Beef, or Leftover Ribs	• Baked Cod or Leftover Ribs • Sautéed Brussels Sprouts	• Broccoli Detox Soup • Side Salad
3	• Broccoli Detox Soup • Sautéed Brussels Sprouts	• Braised Beef & Onions • Kale Crunch	• Wilted Garlic Salad • Roasted Vegetables
4	• Bowl of Soup • Roasted Vegetables	• Baked Salmon • Mixed Greens Salad	• Garbage Stir-Fry • Cup of Broth
5	• Turkey Breakfast Patties • Kale Crunch	• Garbage Stir-Fry • Lemon-Massaged Kale Salad	• Ground Beef or Turkey • Vegetable Medley
6	• Cleansing Smoothie • Vegetable Medley	• Tuna Salad • Soup of Choice	• Sautéed Fennel & Onions • Cauliflower Mashed "Potatoes"
7	• Roast Beef Lettuce Wrap • Sautéed Fennel & Onions	• Garden Salad with Sautéed Veggies	• Vegetable Soup • Side Salad
8	• Berry Green Smoothie • Herbed Zucchini & Carrot Salad	• Vegetable Soup • Salad of Choice	• Braised Green Beans • Pan-Fried Salmon
9	• Rainbow Salad • Bowl of Broth	• Lemon-Massaged Kale Salad • Soup of Choice	• Slow Cooker Turkey Stew
10	• Turkey or Beef Breakfast Patties • Kale Crunch	• Lettuce Wrap with Meat of Choice • Salad of Choice	• French Onion Soup • Braised Green Beans
11	• French Onion Soup • Green Beans	• Baked Mahi-Mahi with Crunchy Fennel Salad	• Kale & Onion Sauté • Cup of Broth
12	• Kale & Onion Sauté • Broccoli Detox Soup	• Garden Salad with Sautéed Onions • Cup of Soup of Choice	• Asian Ground Beef with Mushroom & Broccoli Slaw

Digestive Cleanse Recipes

These recipes serve not only for use during the cleanse; they may also introduce you to new food types, combinations, and cooking processes. The goal is to find some recipes that you will carry forward as staples after the cleanse as well.

Items to Note

- In the Digestive Cleanse Menu Plan on the previous page, you'll see the same dish repeated within the next day or two. This means you can either eat the leftovers from your previous cooking session, or you can make the meal again.

- If your energy drops during the day, make sure to eat more and add protein, like fish or grass-fed meat. For a quick and versatile option, sprinkle some plain collagen powder into any dish.

- Eat at least two to three cups of vegetables at each meal. They should fill a dinner plate.

- If you get deli or other processed meats, make sure they are nitrate free, carrageenan free, and sugar free (less than a gram). Deli meats are high histamine, so avoid if you have histamine issues.

- If you are frequently hungry, eat more fat like olive oil and protein.

- When starting on the cleanse, it can help to make soup. Soup is more filling than other foods because it is a warm liquid. It is also easy to store and heat up. You can add a protein to your leftover soup, either in the soup or on the side. Suggested proteins include a jar of sardines in olive oil or sautéed ground beef.

- Quick protein snack on the go: If you are eating meat and need a clean snack, the Epic and Simply Snackin' meat snacks are a good option.

For Day 1

Bone Broth (make early in cleanse and use again)

Makes 3–4 quarts
Source: Paul Pitchford, Healing with Whole Foods, *3rd edition*

- 2–2½ lbs bones from an organically raised animal
- 2 lbs vegetable/herb scraps or whole veggies
- 2 Tbsp apple cider vinegar (helps release collagen from the animal bones)
- Enough water to cover ingredients

Put all ingredients into a large pot.* Bring to a simmer, remove scum with a slotted spoon, cover, and gently simmer (never boil) for 4 hours. Let cool a bit and strain into glass jars. Refrigerate and use within a week, or freeze. Use alone as a drink or soup, or as a liquid base for other dishes. Fat will settle on the top and should be removed but can be used as cooking fat or discarded.

Slow Cooker Variation: Put all ingredients in a slow cooker and cook on low for 7–8 hours.

*You can cook the broth with some or all of the veggies, and/or wait to add them when making soup.

Why Bone Broth?

The advantage of this animal product is its unique nutrition from the marrow, which is known in China to promote growth and development. There, a broth from broken bones and vegetables is called "longevity soup." One of the vital nutrients in marrow is the omega-3 fatty acid DHA, which is required for the development of the brain, eyes, and other organs in infants.

Historical precedents for this practice exist in most other traditional cultures as well, including Native America, where children were given bones to suck out the marrow.

People who are vegetarian for ethical reasons may see this as not directly involved in taking animal life, since bones that would otherwise be discarded can be obtained.

A word of caution: Avoid animals raised where lead has deposited from auto exhausts or other sources over the years, since lead collects in the bones and marrow of animals. Today more than ever, it is important to know about the sources of your food.

Vegetable Broth from Scraps
Keep a gallon zip-top bag in your freezer, making sure it's handy the next time you are chopping vegetables. Put things like carrot tops and peelings, parsnip peelings, celery ends, and onion skins in the bag.

You can add whatever veggies you like, but a good rule is to stay away from anything with an overpowering taste, like cabbage or broccoli, unless you would like that flavor.

Store the bag of vegetable scraps in your freezer. When it's full, simply add it to the slow cooker, cover the scraps with water, and simmer for 4 hours.

Strain and freeze your broth for whenever you need it. Drink it for a nice warm drink. You can even freeze it in ice cube trays so it's preportioned for when you need smaller amounts.

This simple method should yield two to three quarts of broth that are all homemade and have no preservatives. Plus you are saving money and curbing food waste!

If you do not want to wait for a full bag of scraps, put in whole veggies and then eat or puree them later for a soup.

Basic Soup

Recipe adapted from Dr. Marcus Ettinger

*The vegetables below can be varied! You can mix it up by adding in a big head of kale, collards, a bag of frozen mushrooms, or whatever low-starch veggies you have on hand.

- 2 cloves garlic*
- 1–2 medium onions*
- 1 head cauliflower, chopped*
- 3 medium zucchinis, chopped*
- 4–8 stalks celery, chopped*
- 7 Tbsp fat (lard, olive oil, duck fat)
- 1 quart broth (vegetable and/or bone)
- Seasonings: 1 Tbsp Italian herbs (feel free to try different blends)
- Sea salt to taste

Cook down the garlic and onions in 3 Tbsp of your fat of choice. Then add the rest of the vegetables, broth, and seasonings. After it's done cooking, blend the soup, then add 4 additional Tbsp of your fat. Serve it with your protein of choice (like fish or grass-fed meat). Making two big batches of soup per week will last most of the week and provide several easy meals.

Cleansing Smoothie

- 1½ cups cold water
- ½ cup pea or broccoli sprouts
- ¼ tsp powdered or fresh ginger
- 1 handful mixed greens
- 3 kale leaves (stems removed)
- ½ lemon, juiced
- 1 green apple (avoid if ketogenic)
- ½ cup berries (avoid or use less than ¼ cup if ketogenic)

Add ingredients to a high-speed blender and blend until smooth.

Berry Green Smoothie

- 1 cup water
- 1 handful mixed greens
- 1 tsp green drink powder or liquid chlorophyll
- 1–2 scoops protein powder (collagen or pea protein, about 20 g)
- 2 handfuls fresh or frozen berries (avoid or use less than ¼ cup if ketogenic)

Add ingredients to a high-speed blender and blend until smooth.

Rainbow Salad

- 4–6 oz romaine lettuce
- ½ cup sugar snap peas, cut in half; remove end where stem attached
- 1 beauty heart radish, sliced into discs or grated
- 1 small carrot, sliced into discs or grated (avoid if ketogenic)

Dressing

- 1 Tbsp raw apple cider vinegar
- 4 Tbsp extra-virgin olive oil
- 1 Tbsp shallot or onion, minced
- Sea salt to taste

In a small bowl, mix together vinegar, shallot, salt, and pepper. Allow to sit for a minute or two. Begin whisking ingredients together, then slowly stream in oil while continuing to whisk. Set dressing aside.

Divide greens between two large salad bowls, and sprinkle vegetables over them evenly. Top with dressing and serve.

Lettuce Wraps with Meat of Choice

- Nitrate-free, carrageenan-free deli meats (roast beef, turkey, etc.)
- Sliced vegetables and herbs (sprouts, pesto, olive oil, fresh basil, cucumbers, radishes, sautéed mushrooms, etc.)

- Large leaves of romaine lettuce or collard greens

- A sauce of your choice from the Sauces and Dip Recipes section (mayo, pesto, etc.).

Lay the meat, vegetables, and sauce out on a large flat leaf of your greens and roll it up into a handheld wrap. Repeat until you are full!

Slow Cooker Ribs

- 1–2 large racks of ribs (thaw if necessary)
- Sea salt and any fresh or dried seasonings (cumin, oregano, etc.)

Season the ribs. Place in the slow cooker on low for 6–8 hours. Enjoy with fresh salad and/or roasted vegetables.

Fried or Grilled Zucchini

Serves 2–4

- 1½ lbs zucchini, trimmed and sliced lengthwise in ½" strips
- 2 Tbsp olive oil
- Sea salt
- Apple cider vinegar
- Handful of basil leaves, cut thinly

Lay the zucchini on a baking sheet and brush both sides with oil. Then season liberally with salt.

Cook the squash on the gas grill set on medium heat for about 8–10 minutes total. (Flip once at the 4-minute mark.) Or fry on the stove top in olive oil until browned, flipping after a few minutes.

Before serving, if desired, drizzle with vinegar and sprinkle with fresh basil or any other seasoning you would like. Leftovers could be used for another meal or put in a wrap or salad.

For Day 2

Baked Cod

Preheat oven to 400° (or set toaster oven to 400°). Season the cod with sea salt and other spices to taste. Drizzle olive oil on the pan and on top of the fillet. Bake for 15–20 minutes depending on the size of the fish.

Sautéed Brussels Sprouts

- 1 lb brussels sprouts, halved (remove any discolored leaves)
- 1 small onion, sliced
- 2 Tbsp olive oil
- 1 tsp garlic, powder or fresh
- Sea salt to taste

Heat olive oil in large pan/wok for a minute on medium heat. Add brussels sprouts, onions, garlic, and salt to the pan and sauté until desired texture.

Broccoli Detox Soup

Serves 2–3

- 2 Tbsp olive oil
- 1 bunch broccoli, chopped (remove skin of stems)
- 1 cup greens (arugula, kale, collards, bok choy)
- 1 large carrot, chopped (leave out if ketogenic)
- 1 onion, chopped
- 2 garlic cloves, chopped
- 2–3 cups water or broth
- Sea salt

Add oil to a large pot over medium heat. Add broccoli, greens, carrot, onion, and garlic to the pot and stir for about 3 minutes. Cover with water or broth and add sea salt to taste.

Simmer the vegetables for about 5 minutes until they are cooked but not too soft. Either leave the soup unblended or blend the soup using an immersion blender or a high-speed blender until smooth.

Side Salad

This can be whatever you like. Start with a lettuce, spinach, or greens mix. Add whatever fresh vegetables you have on hand: celery, radishes, onions, et cetera. Top with olive oil and lemon juice or apple cider vinegar. Experiment by adding different herbs, fresh minced garlic, or a dressing from the Dressing and Sauce section.

For Day 3

Braised Beef & Onions

Serves 4
Adapted from Epicurious.com

- 1 boneless beef chuck pot roast (2 lbs, about 1½" thick)
- ¾ lb onions, halved lengthwise, then thinly sliced lengthwise (3 cups)
- 3 large garlic cloves, finely chopped
- 1 Tbsp fresh flat-leaf parsley, finely chopped
- Sea salt ground pepper
- 1–2 tsp cumin powder, optional
- Water or broth to cover roast halfway

Put oven rack in middle position and preheat oven to 275°. Pat meat dry and season.

Spread half the onions and half the garlic in a 13" × 9" roasting pan with a cover and arrange meat on top. Spread remaining onions and garlic over meat. Cover pan and roast, turning meat over after 1 hour, until meat is very tender, about 3 hours total. Slice meat across the grain and sprinkle with parsley. Serve with onions and pan juices.

Slow cooker option: Prepare meat as above. Place in slow cooker with onions and garlic. Cover and set on Low for 8 hours.

You may not need as much water or broth with this method. (I typically do not use any liquid in a slow cooker unless the roast is very lean.)

Kale Crunch (Kale Chips)

Yields 2–4 cups
From Mollie Katzen's Vegetable Heaven

- A little olive oil for the baking tray
- 1 giant bunch fresh kale, stemmed and minced (about 1 lb)
- Sea salt to taste

Try these "chips" for snacking or for sprinkling on any savory dish. Baking kale is an interesting process. First, the leaves become bright green and soften, and then they begin to turn crisp. In between, they go through a chewy-crisp stage, which is also delicious. Therefore, the baking time is flexible. Just keep checking the kale until it is done the way you like it.

Preheat oven to 350°. Line a large baking tray with foil, then brush it with oil. Add the kale, spreading it out as much as possible. Bake for 10 minutes, mixing it up once or twice during that time. Bake for 10–15 minutes longer, stirring occasionally, until it's as crisp as you like it. The kale will continue to shrink and crispen the longer it bakes. When it's baked to your liking, remove from the oven, and let the kale cool on the tray.

To ensure you have leftovers, try doubling the recipe. Store leftover kale in a brown paper bag with a paper towel inside (to absorb the moisture).

Wilted Garlic Salad

- 1 Tbsp olive oil
- 1 clove garlic, minced
- 1 lb swiss chard or other green of choice
- Sea salt

Warm oil in large skillet over medium heat. Add garlic and stir until lightly browned, about 1 minute. Add greens and toss until just wilted, 2–4 minutes. Season to taste with salt or other seasonings.

Roasted Vegetables with Rosemary

Serves 3–4

You can roast any number of vegetables with some olive oil in the oven. Onions, shiitake mushrooms, zucchini, brussels sprouts, and cabbage are just a few examples that are very filling and delicious when roasted.

- 3 lbs vegetables
- 4+ cloves garlic, finely chopped
- 3 Tbsp raw apple cider vinegar (optional)
- 3 Tbsp cold-pressed olive oil
- 1 Tbsp fresh rosemary
- 1 tsp each dried herbs such as parsley, oregano, basil, etc.
- 2 tsp sea salt

Preheat oven to 375°. Chop vegetables into ½" cubes. In a small bowl, combine olive oil, vinegar, rosemary, other herbs, and sea salt to make a marinade.

Place veggies on a baking dish and toss with the marinade. Then place veggies in a single layer in the dish. Roast in oven for 40–60 minutes or until tender and light brown. You may need to stir the veggies after approximately 20 minutes. Add garlic when stirring at 20 minutes.

Serve alone or on a bed of fresh greens such as spinach, mustard greens, lettuce, or the sautéed greens from beets, turnips, and carrots.

For Day 4

Baked Salmon

Preheat oven to 400° (or set toaster oven to 400°). Season the salmon with sea salt and other spices to taste. Dill is good also. Bake for 15–20 minutes depending on the size of the fish.

Mixed Greens Salad

Use greens of your choice with chopped radishes, cucumbers, peas, or any nonstarchy vegetable you feel like adding. You may top with caramelized or sautéed veggies for a different texture.

Garbage Stir-Fry

From nomnompaleo.com

This recipe makes use of whatever wilting veggies are in the fridge or freezer. There are no set measurements, and it's never the same twice. Basic elements include:

• Nonstarchy veggies (greens, broccoli, mushrooms, etc.), chopped
• ½–1 cup onions, leeks, or shallots, diced
• 2 Tbsp of your favorite cooking fat (olive oil, lard, duck fat, etc.)
• 1–2 Tbsp of your favorite seasoning
• Sea salt

Heat cooking fat in a pan. Add the onions and cook until fragrant. Add the rest of the veggies and cook until desired texture. Mix in your favorite seasoning and top with salt to taste!

For Day 5

Turkey Breakfast Patties

Serves 3–4

• 1 lb ground turkey, grass-fed ground beef, or free-range pork

- ¼ tsp each cumin, ginger, marjoram, turmeric, thyme, and cayenne pepper (omit if avoiding nightshade foods)
- ½ tsp each basil, oregano, and sage
- 1½ tsp sea salt
- Optional: 1 small onion

If adding onion, chop and sauté and set aside to cool. Then mix all ingredients and chill for 15–30 minutes. Remove from the refrigerator and form into patties. If not using onions, mix all ingredients together and form into 3 or 4 patties.

To freeze: Before cooking, store in an airtight container using parchment paper between each patty, or store in separate containers to pull out for using one at a time. Bake in the oven or sauté in olive oil.

Lemon-Massaged Kale Salad

Serves 4

- 1 bunch kale, thinly sliced
- ½ bunch parsley
- Juice from 1 lemon
- 1 garlic clove, minced
- 2 Tbsp extra-virgin olive oil
- Sea salt

Add all ingredients in a large bowl. Use your bare hands to massage the salad together until the kale is soft and wilted. It should turn a dark green color. Feel free to add other veggies.

Vegetable Medley

Serves 4

- 4 Tbsp olive oil (enough to cover bottom of pan)
- 2 zucchini, diced
- 2 yellow squash, diced

- 2 cups asparagus, diced
- 1 cup fresh mushrooms, sliced
- 1 small red onion, diced
- 3–4 cloves of garlic, minced (4 heaping Tbsp)
- 4 tsp dried thyme
- 1 pinch cayenne (or 1 Tbsp crushed red pepper. Omit if avoiding nightshade family)
- 1 lemon
- Sea salt to taste

Heat olive oil in a saucepan. Add garlic and asparagus and sauté over high heat to sear the greens. Stir asparagus frequently as not to burn. Add thyme, sea salt, and optional cayenne. Then add the rest of the veggies and simmer for 20–25 min. Upon serving, squeeze lemon juice over veggies.

For Day 6

Tuna Salad

Open can or bag of low-mercury yellowfin or skipjack tuna and drain. Mix with homemade mayo (see Dressing and Sauce Recipe section) or drizzle olive oil and apple cider vinegar into bowl with tuna. Serve on top of a large salad or in large lettuce leaves as a roll-up.

Sautéed Fennel & Onions

- 1 fennel bulb
- 1 medium onion
- Olive oil
- Sea salt

Heat oil in a sauté pan on medium heat. Add fennel slices and cook until they are soft and the onions clear. Salt to taste.

Cauliflower Mashed "Potatoes"

From nomnompaleo.com

- 1 head cauliflower, roughly chopped
- 1–2 garlic cloves, sliced
- Sea salt
- 2 Tbsp olive oil

Steam the cauliflower and garlic for about 8–10 minutes on medium high. Add a little salt while steaming. Once the florets are soft, put everything into a colander and let it drain.

Put everything into a box grater/food processor with olive oil. Process everything until smooth.

If you want the texture more like rice, put big flowerets in the food processor first and pulse to the texture of rice. Sauté the cauliflower for 3 minutes. Add the minced garlic and sauté for another 3–5 minutes.

For Day 7

Vegetable Soup

Serves 4–5

- ½ cup olive oil
- 1 large onion, chopped
- 3 stalks celery, chopped
- 2 carrots, diced (avoid if ketogenic)
- 6 cloves garlic, minced
- 2–3 quarts broth
- 1 tsp thyme
- 1 Tbsp Italian seasoning
- 1 tsp sea salt
- 2 bay leaves

- 3 cups cabbage, finely chopped
- 2 cups zucchini, chopped
- ½ cup green beans, chopped

Sauté onion, celery, carrots, and garlic in 2–3 Tbsp olive oil until tender. Add seasonings and broth, and simmer for 15 minutes. Add cabbage, zucchini, and green beans, then the rest of the olive oil.

Simmer until veggies are done to your liking. Slow simmering brings out the flavor of the ingredients.

For Day 8

Herbed Zucchini Salad

Serves 4

- 2 large zucchini, spiralized (or use a vegetable peeler)
- 1 large carrot, shredded (avoid if ketogenic)
- 2 Tbsp olive oil
- 1 garlic clove, minced
- 1 tsp dill, fresh or dried
- 5 mint leaves, torn
- ½ lemon, juiced
- Sea salt

Add all ingredients into a large bowl. Mix thoroughly.

Braised Green Beans

- 1 Tbsp olive oil
- 1 small onion, chopped
- 1 lb fresh green beans
- 2 garlic cloves, minced
- 2/3 cup vegetable broth

Warm a large sauté pan over medium-high heat. Add 1 Tbsp olive oil. When the pan is hot, add the chopped onion. Sauté 2–3 minutes, then add your green beans and garlic and sauté another minute. Add broth, cover the pan with a lid, and steam for about 5 minutes. Then remove the lid and sauté until most of the broth has evaporated.

For Day 9

Slow Cooker Turkey Stew

Adapted from Peter J. D'Adamo's Eat Right 4 Your Type *cookbook*

- 2 tsp olive oil
- 1 lb turkey breast
- 2 cups diced onion
- 2 cups diced carrots (or parsnips after Digestive Cleanse; avoid if ketogenic)
- 4 cups red kale, torn
- 2 large sprigs fresh rosemary
- 4 large sprigs fresh thyme
- 1 cup water
- 1 cup broth

Preheat slow cooker to medium heat. Heat olive oil in a large skillet over medium heat, and brown turkey breast on all sides. Remove turkey from the pan and set aside.

In the same skillet, add onion and carrots, sautéing 3–4 minutes. Add vegetables to the bottom of the slow cooker. Place the turkey breast on top of vegetables, then add rosemary and thyme.
Pour water and stock in the bottom of the skillet to deglaze, scraping up all the bits. Pour liquid and bits over the turkey in the slow cooker and cover.

Let cook 1 hour, then add the kale and cook 1 additional hour.

For Day 10

French Onion Soup

Serves 4

- 4 Tbsp olive oil (or more as needed)
- 3 medium onions, thinly sliced
- 4 cups vegetable or bone broth
- 2 Tbsp chopped fresh thyme or 1 tsp dried
- 2 Tbsp chopped parsley or 1 tsp dried
- 1 bay leaf
- Sea salt to taste

Heat the oil in a large casserole or stockpot over medium-high heat. Add the onions. Cook them, stirring occasionally, until they become a deep mahogany brown. It will take some time to achieve this dark color. Add broth to keep onions from burning. Stir in broth, parsley, thyme, and bay leaf and bring to a boil. Reduce the heat to a simmer and cook for 10 minutes. Remove the bay leaf and season with sea salt.

For Day 11

Baked Mahi-Mahi with Crunchy Fennel Salad

Serves 2
Adapted from Peter J. D'Adamo's Eat Right 4 Your Type *cookbook*

- 1 lb mahi-mahi
- ⅛ tsp ground coriander
- 1 tsp fresh lemon zest
- Sea salt to taste

Crunchy Fennel Salad

- 2 tsp chopped fresh parsley

- 2 tsp olive oil
- 1 tsp lemon zest
- 2 tsp lemon juice
- 1–2 cups thinly sliced fennel
- Sea salt to taste

Preheat oven to 350°. Season mahi-mahi with coriander, lemon zest, and sea salt. Bake for 12–15 minutes, or until fish is flaky and white. While fish bakes, whisk together parsley, olive oil, sea salt to taste, lemon zest, and juice in a bowl. Add fennel and toss to combine. Plate fish, top with fennel salad, and serve immediately.

Kale and Onion Sauté

- 2–3 Tbsp olive oil
- 1 bunch kale, stems and leaves separated and chopped
- 1 large sweet red onion
- 3 cloves garlic, chopped
- Juice of ½ lemon

Put oil in a pan and set at medium heat. Place kale stems in the pan and cook for 5 minutes. Add the kale leaves and onion to the pan. Add the garlic cloves and lemon juice. Cook to desired tenderness (about 10 minutes).

For Day 12

Asian Ground Beef and Mushroom with Broccoli Slaw

From nomnompaleo.com

- 1 lb grass-fed organic ground beef
- ½ lb mushrooms, thinly sliced (cremini, white button, etc.)
- 1 small onion, roughly chopped
- 1–2 cups broccoli, chopped

- ½ cup carrots, shredded (avoid if ketogenic)
- 3 cloves garlic, minced
- 2 scallions, thinly sliced
- Handful cilantro, coarsely chopped
- 2 Tbsp olive oil
- 1–2 Tbsp apple cider vinegar
- 1 Tbsp sea salt
- Red butter lettuce leaves

Finely chop the onion (by hand or food processor). Pulverizing the onions helps moisten the meat and it cooks much faster.

Then put the onions into the skillet with oil and sauté on medium heat until translucent. Add the sliced mushrooms and a pinch of salt. When the onions and mushrooms have released the excess moisture, add the minced garlic cloves and stir everything for 30 seconds.

Next, add the ground beef and stir until there are no large clumps and it is no longer pink. Add the apple cider vinegar and more salt, and taste for seasoning. Once the meat is cooked and seasoned, add the broccoli and carrots and stir everything around to soften the veggies a bit. Finally, add the scallions and cilantro and mix to distribute everything evenly. Serve the beef-and-veggie mixture on red butter lettuce leaves.

Additional Digestive Cleanse Recipes

Taco Salad

- 2 lbs ground beef or other leftover meat
- 1–2 tsp cumin
- 1–2 tsp sea salt
- 2 stalks celery, chopped
- 1–2 radishes, grated
- ¼ bunch cilantro, finely chopped
- Fresh greens (a few big handfuls)
- Fresh sprouts (a few Tbsp)
- 1 cucumber, cubed
- 1–2 carrots, grated (optional; avoid if ketogenic)
- ½ beet, grated (optional; avoid if ketogenic)

Brown the ground beef on a skillet over medium heat. When it is almost cooked through, add the cumin and sea salt and stir well. Make a salad on your plate starting with the greens on the bottom and piling up the veggies. Put the meat on top and add a vinaigrette dressing (see the Dressing and Sauce Recipe section).

Sautéed Collard Greens & Onions

Serves 3

- 1 bunch collard greens, stems and leaves separated and chopped
- 1 large onion, chopped into large chunks
- 2 medium carrots (avoid if ketogenic), sliced into discs
- Olive oil
- Sea salt

Pour enough olive oil into a sauté pan to cover the bottom. Heat at medium heat and add the stems. Season with sea salt or your choice of seasoning. Cook for 5–7 minutes. Add the rest of the veggies to the pan and sauté for another 10–15 minutes.

Critter Cleanse Recipes

Onion-Wilted Spinach Salad with Avocado

Serves 4 to 6
From Mollie Katzen's Vegetable Heaven

Fresh spinach becomes tender when combined with warmed ingredients, causing it to wilt slightly. This recipe tastes best immediately after it has been assembled, when the onion is still warm. The avocado is delicious but optional.

- 3 Tbsp fresh lemon juice
- 3 Tbsp olive oil
- 2 cups onions, sliced into thick rings
- 1½ tsp cumin seeds
- ½ lb spinach, cleaned and stemmed
- Sea salt
- 1 small ripe avocado (optional)

Pour the lemon juice onto a plate. Peel and slice the avocado, then coat the avocado slices in the lemon juice. Set aside.

Heat the olive oil in a medium-sized skillet. When it is hot, add the onion rings and cook over medium-high heat for 3–5 minutes. Sprinkle in the cumin seeds and cook for just a minute longer.

Add the hot onion and cumin to the spinach and toss until thoroughly mixed. The spinach will begin to wilt upon contact. To speed this process along—and to be sure you include every last drop of the flavorful oil—you can add some of the spinach directly to the pan and swish it around a little, then return it to the bowl. Toss while adding salt.

Gently mix in the avocado, including all the lemon juice. Add optional cooked protein and serve right away.

Jicama Coconut Rice

From www.goneraw.com

- 3 large jicamas, peeled
- 3 Tbsp olive oil
- 2 Tbsp parsley, chopped (optional)
- ½ tsp finely ground sea salt (or to taste)
- 2 cups organic dried coconut (unsweetened), shredded

Cut the jicama into small chunks and use a food processor on pulse to chop it into rice-sized grains. Place in large serving bowl. Add the rest of the ingredients and mix well. Serve cold or slightly warmed up.

Non-Ketogenic Recipes

Curried Carrot Bok Choy Soup

Serves 4

Not ketogenic (too starchy)

- 3 lbs medium carrots, chopped
- 1 medium bunch of bok choy, chopped
- 1 red onion
- 2 Tbsp garlic, minced
- Olive oil
- 2 quarts vegetable broth
- Herb and garlic seasoning
- 2 Tbsp cumin
- 1 Tbsp red curry seasoning
- Sea salt

Cover the bottom of a large pot with olive oil and add carrots, onion, bok choy, and seasonings (garlic, cumin, curry, garlic). Over medium-high heat, stir constantly and cook until tender. Add broth to cover the vegetables, bring to a boil, and then simmer for 10 minutes. Season to taste. Add extra olive oil to give it a heartier taste. (Note: To save time, you can heat up the broth in a separate pot while you sauté the vegetables. Then combine the hot broth with the tender vegetables and simmer for 10 minutes).

Roasted Squash

Not ketogenic (too starchy)

- 1 very large winter squash or 2 small ones
- Extra-virgin coconut oil
- Sea salt
- Cinnamon, if desired

Preheat oven to 400°. Chop squash into a few large pieces and clean out the seeds. Put a dollop of coconut oil in the base of each piece and sprinkle with salt, cinnamon, and any other seasonings you like. Add ½ cup water in the bottom of the pan. Place in a deep pan and cover with lid. Bake until soft, about an hour.

Spaghetti Squash with Browned Ground Meat

Serves 3–4
Not ketogenic (too starchy)

- 1 large spaghetti squash
- 1–2 lbs ground beef, bison, or chicken
- 8 oz fresh mushrooms, sliced
- 1 zucchini, diced
- 1 yellow squash, sliced
- 1 red onion, diced
- 3 heaping Tbsp fresh garlic, minced
- 1 tsp Italian seasoning
- 1 tsp thyme
- 1 Tbsp crushed red pepper (omit if avoiding nightshade family))
- 1 tsp basil
- 1 tsp oregano
- 3 Tbsp olive oil

- Sea salt to taste
- *Optional:* Top with pesto sauce (see Dressing and Sauce Recipes)

Preheat the oven to 450° and place spaghetti squash in a large saucepan. Add enough water to cover the bottom of the pan. Poke a few holes in the squash with a fork to allow steam to escape. Cover and place the squash in the oven and cook for 45 minutes to 1 hour (time may vary depending on size of squash.)

While the spaghetti squash is cooking, heat olive oil in a large saucepan and add all the veggies and seasonings. Sauté the veggies 20–25 minutes or until they are soft. If desired, add pesto and heat on low with veggies. Once spaghetti squash is cooked, cut in the middle and fork out the squash onto a serving dish. (It should look like noodles inside.) Place sauce over "noodles."

Brown the meat separately and spoon over noodles.

Parsnip Puree

Serves 4
Adapted from Ming Tsai's Blue Ginger *cookbook*
A sweet and hearty entrée or dessert. Not ketogenic (too starchy)

- 4 cups (about 1½ lbs) parsnips (peeling optional), 1" pieces
- 5 garlic cloves, peeled
- Sea salt and black pepper
- 4 Tbsp olive oil
- 1 Tbsp honey (optional)

Combine the parsnips and garlic in a large saucepan, then add water to cover and a pinch of salt. Bring to a boil, reduce the heat, and simmer until the point of a knife inserted into the parsnips meets no resistance, about 25 minutes. Drain, transfer to a food processor, and puree. Add the rest of the ingredients. Pulse to blend. Keep warm.

Purifying Beet Salad

Serves 5–6
Beets are a starchy vegetable and normally avoided during the Digestive Cleanse but may be taken in some cases for their support of the liver.

- 1 cup raw beets, shredded
- 2 Tbsp extra-virgin olive oil
- ½ lemon, juiced

Combine all ingredients, cover, and store in the refrigerator. Use 1–2 Tbsp per meal to enhance salads and grain dishes.

Roasted Root Vegetable Soup

Serves 4
Not ketogenic (too starchy)

- 10 large carrots or other root vegetables, chopped into finger-length pieces
- 2 medium onions, peeled and coarsely chopped
- 3–7 cloves garlic, peeled
- 3 Tbsp olive oil
- 4–6 cups hot water or vegetable broth
- 3 Tbsp dried basil
- Seasonings: sea salt, dash of olive oil and dash of apple cider vinegar, and cayenne pepper or paprika

Preheat oven to 375°. Chop carrots, onions, garlic, and any other vegetables you would like to put in soup (celeriac, turnips, etc.) and place on a baking dish with the olive oil and cover.

Bake until carrots are soft to your liking (make take 40–60 minutes). The longer you roast, the sweeter the carrots will get. About 10 minutes prior to removing the carrots from the oven, heat the water or broth on the stove until boiling.

When carrots and water are done, combine both in a food processor or blender. If you have a small blender, you may need to do this in two batches or more. Add less water for a thicker stew, more for a thin puree. Taste your soup and decide what seasonings to try. A little vinegar will give it a "zip." More oil will make it "heavier." Experiment with this recipe using other veggies like cabbage, brussels sprouts, or squash.

Butternut Squash Soup

Serves 2 to 4
Not ketogenic (too starchy)

- 1 large butternut or delicate squash
- 2 zucchinis
- 1 large onion
- 1 Tbsp fresh ginger
- 1 quart filtered water (for thicker soup, use ½ quart)
- Cinnamon, black pepper, onion powder (all to taste)

Chop vegetables and ginger and simmer with spices in water until soft. Puree in a blender or food processor.

Roasted Carrot "Fries"

Not ketogenic (too starchy)

- 2–3 large carrots
- 1–2 Tbsp olive oil, coconut oil, or lard
- Sea salt and ground pepper

Cut the carrots into "fry" shapes using a knife or the larger shredder setting on a mandolin. Next, toss the fries with the oil, salt, and pepper. Bake at 450° for 40–45 minutes or until they are slightly browned.

CKG Smoothie (Carrot, Kale, Ginger)

Serves 4
Adapted from Peter J. D'Adamo's Eat Right 4 Your Type *cookbook*
Not ketogenic (too starchy)

- 4 large carrots (avoid if ketogenic)
- 1 bunch of kale
- 1 3" piece fresh ginger, peeled
- ½ lemon
- 4 Granny Smith apples (avoid if ketogenic)

This could be blended into a smoothie (in a blender) or juiced (run each item through the juicer one at a time).

Kidney Cleanse Recipes

White Bean Preparation

Instructions for cooking dry beans for maximum digestibility:

1. Rinse the beans well and remove any rocks and bad-looking beans.

2. Cover the beans with filtered water and let soak overnight. To speed up this process, bring the water to a boil, then turn off the heat and let the beans sit for at least 4–6 hours.

3. Rinse the beans thoroughly and discard soak water.

4. Cover the beans with fresh filtered water and place on the stove. Do not salt the beans at this point (or at all during a Kidney Cleanse); this will make it harder to soften them. Cover the pot and bring the beans to a boil. (You may put a bit of kombucha seaweed in with the beans to help digest the proteins and starches.)

5. If the beans foam when boiling, turn down the heat and remove the foam with a slotted spoon and discard. Removing the foam will enhance the digestibility of the beans.

6. Allow the pot to simmer for 2–6 hours or more until the beans are soft. The older and bigger the bean, the longer it will take to cook. Therefore, times suggested in recipes are not always reliable.

7. When the beans are soft, add 1 Tbsp apple cider vinegar and simmer for 10 more minutes on the stove to break down additional proteins and starches.

8. Remove the beans from the heat, and strain.

9. Add the beans into your favorite recipe! Beans digest best in combination with raw, nonstarchy vegetables. (Think bean dip and veggie sticks, or toss beans in with salad).

Bean Soup with Kale

Serves 7–8

- 1 Tbsp olive oil
- 8 garlic cloves, minced
- 1 medium yellow onion, chopped
- 4 cups raw kale, chopped
- 4 cups vegetable broth
- 3 cups cooked beans, such as white or cannellini
- 4 plum tomatoes, chopped (omit if avoiding nightshade family))
- 2 tsp dried Italian seasoning (or 1 tsp each dried thyme and rosemary)
- 1 cup fresh parsley, minced
- Sea salt

In a large pot, heat olive oil. Add garlic and onion, and sauté until soft. Add kale and sauté, stirring until wilted. Add 3 cups of broth, 2 cups of beans, the optional tomatoes, and all herbs. Simmer for 5 minutes.

In a blender or food processor, mix the remaining beans and broth until smooth. Stir into soup to thicken. Simmer for 5–10 minutes. Ladle into bowls and sprinkle with parsley for color.

Fresh Herb Bean Spread

- 3 cloves garlic
- 3 cups cooked beans, white or cannellini
- 3 Tbsp lime juice
- 2 Tbsp olive oil
- 2 Tbsp fresh basil
- 1 Tbsp fresh thyme
- 1 tsp sea salt

Blend beans, garlic, lime juice, and oil in food processor. Add herbs until coarsely chopped. Salt to taste. Serve with fresh vegetables.

Basic Chia Pudding

Serves 2–3

- ¾ cup chia seeds
- 2 cups coconut milk
- ¼ tsp cinnamon or spice of choice
- Stevia and vanilla extract to taste (not on cleanse)

Simply mix the ingredients together, and let them rest for a few moments. Stir the mix well with a fork every five minutes or so. At first, it will seem far too runny, but over the course of 30 minutes, the chia seeds will plump up till the mixture resembles tapioca pudding.

Liver Cleanse Recipes

Nut & Seed Pâté

Makes a substantial amount, so you may want to halve the recipe amounts

- 1 cup almonds, soaked 12–48 hours and blanched
- 1 cup pumpkin seeds, soaked 6–8 hours and rinsed
- 3 stalks celery, finely chopped
- 1 small leek, finely chopped
- 1–2 tsp powdered kelp
- Sea salt to taste
- 2 Tbsp lemon juice

Using a Champion juicer (with the solid plate) or food processor, process almonds and pumpkin seeds until ground smooth. Add celery, leek, lemon juice, kelp, and salt and mix well. Serve with veggies.

Homemade Applesauce

Serves 5–6
Adapted from Peter J. D'Adamo's Eat Right 4 Your Type *cookbook*
Not ketogenic (too sweet)

- 4 Granny Smith apples, diced (about 2 cups)
- 1 cinnamon stick
- ½ cup apple juice
- ½ cup frozen raspberries

Combine all ingredients: apples, cinnamon stick, apple juice, and raspberries in a saucepan set over medium heat. Cook 30 minutes, or until apples no longer hold their shape. Stir occasionally, remove from heat, and serve warm or chilled.

Recipes for After the Cleanse

Slow Cooker Chicken

- 1 whole organic, free-range chicken
- Sea salt
- Lemon
- Other seasonings as desired

Pull out any neck/organs that may be inside the chicken (you can use these in other recipes—look up preparing organ meats, making broth, etc.). Rub the chicken's outside with sea salt and any other desired seasonings. Add the lemon to the inside of the chicken if you wish.

Place the chicken in the slow cooker on low for 3–4 hours. Use a meat thermometer to check the internal temperature is 180–190° before removing. Let chicken cool in the slow cooker for 30 minutes and then use a fork and carving knife to carve.

Spinach & Cilantro Egg Scramble

- 4 eggs
- 1 Tbsp olive oil
- 2 cups spinach
- ½ bunch cilantro, chopped
- 2 scallions
- 1 tsp oregano
- Sea salt and pepper

Add eggs to a mixing bowl and mix with a fork. Set to the side.

Add oil to a hot pan. When the oil is melted, add spinach, cilantro, scallion, oregano, sea salt, and pepper. Sauté until the spinach is wilted (2–3 minutes). Add the eggs and mix with the vegetables. Cook to your liking.

Lemon Ginger Sweet Potatoes

Not ketogenic (too starchy)

- 1 medium sweet potato
- ½ lemon, sliced in half
- Dash powdered ginger
- 1–2 tsp coconut oil
- Sea salt and pepper

Preheat oven to 400°. Line a baking sheet with parchment paper. Poke the sweet potato with a fork 3–4 times to allow for even cooking. Place the sweet potato on the baking sheet and roast for 30–45 minutes. The amount of time needed to roast the sweet potatoes all the way through depends on the size of the potato.

You will know the sweet potato is done when you can slide a butter knife through the center without resistance. Once the sweet potato is done, slice it lengthwise down the center. Top with a squeeze of lemon, powdered ginger, coconut oil, sea salt, and pepper.

Kale & Sweet Potato Hash

From www.elizabethrider.com/kale-sweet-potato-hash-recipe/
Not ketogenic (too starchy)

- 2 Tbsp extra-virgin olive oil, divided
- 3 cups sweet potato, grated (from 1 medium sweet potato, skin off for easier digestion)
- 1½ cups kale, chopped (from 5–7 destemmed leaves)
- Sea salt

Sauté the kale in ½ Tbsp oil (you can do this in a separate pan while the potatoes cook.)

While the skillet preheats, grate the sweet potato with a box grater or in a food processor with the grating attachment. Pat dry with paper towels to remove excess moisture.

Add 1½ Tbsp oil to the pan and let it heat up for 10–15 seconds. Add the potatoes with a big pinch of sea salt (season to taste).

Toss the potatoes in the oil with a spatula, then spread evenly. Let cook untouched for 2 minutes. Flip the potatoes and cook until slightly crispy, about another 2 minutes.

Turn off the heat; add the kale and toss together. Remove from the pan and serve.

Sautéed Peas & Carrots

Not ketogenic (too starchy)

Quick option: Cut open a bag of frozen peas and carrots and warm on the stove top in olive oil and add sea salt.

Healthier option: Dice up some carrots and take the peas out of sugar snap pea pods. Add to warm olive oil. Add sea salt and sauté for 5 minutes or to desired tenderness. Watch or peas will get hard if overcooked.

Spicy Collards

Serves 3
From Peter J. D'Adamo's Eat Right 4 Your Type *cookbook*

- 2 tsp olive oil
- ½ cup diced shallots
- 4–5 slices turkey bacon, finely diced
- ½ tsp chili powder or paprika
- 1 bunch collard greens, chopped
- 2 cups black-eyed peas or adzuki beans, cooked (optional)
- Sea salt

Melt olive oil in a large skillet or wok over medium heat. Add shallots, collard stems, and bacon, and sauté until bacon is crispy, about 4–5 minutes (or bake bacon ahead of time to crisp it up if you like it crispy).

Season with spices and add collard greens. Cook 10–12 minutes, until collards are tender and slightly wilted. Add black-eyed peas and cook an additional 3–4 minutes to warm beans.

Garlic & Herb Squash

Not ketogenic (too starchy)

- 2 acorn squashes
- 1 cup water
- 2 Tbsp ghee (clarified butter)
- Sea salt
- 1 Tbsp garlic powder
- 1 Tbsp Italian seasoning

Preheat oven to 350°. Poke a few holes in squash with a large fork or knife and place squash in large baking pan. Add water and place in oven for 45 minutes or until tender. Remove from oven and let cool for 15 minutes.

Cut open the squash and remove the seeds (discard or roast them later). Scoop out the remaining squash into a pan. Add ghee, sea salt, garlic powder, seasonings. Mix well over low heat on the stove top. Stir until smooth.

To roast the seeds: Rinse seeds and place in baking pan. Cover with olive oil and sprinkle with sea salt, garlic powder, and herb seasoning. Place in oven until golden brown (approximately 10–20 min—watch carefully!)

Whole-Grain Waffles

Makes four 5" waffles
Not ketogenic (too starchy)

A great introduction to grains after avoiding them during the cleanses, this recipe includes soaking, rinsing, blending, then cooking the grains into waffles. Try this about 5 or more days after the Liver Cleanse.

- 1 cup millet
- 1 cup rice
- ½ cup coconut milk
- ½ banana
- Sea salt
- Seasonings to your taste (nutmeg, coriander, and/or cinnamon)

First day: Place millet and rice in a medium bowl and cover with filtered water. Loosely cover with a kitchen towel and let stand on the counter overnight. If something prevents you from using it the next morning, just pour off the water, add fresh water, and place it, covered, in the refrigerator for up to 2 days. For a lighter waffle, try buckwheat and/or quinoa.

Next day: Drain and rinse the millet and place it in a blender. Add the coconut milk and banana, and salt to taste.

Process into a thick batter with a blender. Add more coconut milk or water to make the desired consistency, if necessary. Pour batter onto a hot waffle iron, close and bake according to manufacturer's directions.

Raw Cacao Pudding

Serves 2

Not ketogenic (too sweet)

- 2 bananas
- 1 avocado
- 4 Tbsp raw cacao powder
- 1 tsp vanilla

Add the ingredients to a food processor or blender. Once blended, add mixture to a serving bowl, cover, and chill in the refrigerator for at least 30 minutes. Enjoy as is or topped with berries.

Note: If you get a big energy drop after this treat, you can't do cocoa yet.

Dressing and Sauce Recipes

Most salad dressings have an oil base and will include vinegar or lemon, in addition to other seasonings. Olive oil is the most commonly used base, but Udo's and flaxseed oil are also good choices.

Ingesting four tablespoons of olive oil or flaxseed oil daily aids in the digestive process, which allows food to be broken down and nutrients absorbed. These oils help reduce inflammation in the body and are good for the liver and gallbladder. Feel free to add fresh vegetables to the dressing too. Adding fresh garlic, parsley, cilantro, or basil makes a pesto dressing when blended.

When using these recipes, be creative! Add a little bit of this or that to your liking. This activity can only improve your ability to create a version of your own. The best salad greens to use are the deepest greens you can find, such as arugula, escarole, spinach, romaine, baby leaf, kale, or an organic blend of all of these combined. You could also sauté veggies and cover them in a dressing.

Vinaigrette
- 5 Tbsp olive oil or Udo's oil
- 2–3 Tbsp apple cider vinegar or lemon juice
- 1 Tbsp fresh garlic, minced
- 1 Tbsp Italian seasoning
- Optional: ½ cucumber, peeled, chopped, and blended with the other ingredients, or fresh herbs (parsley, cilantro, basil, etc.)

Mix in a bowl until blended. For a creamy version, add to blender for 30 seconds or until desired thickness.

Whole Roasted Garlic (& Sauce)

- 1 head garlic per person

Preheat the oven to 400°. Chop the top of the garlic head off so that just the tips of the pale cloves inside are exposed. Leave the papery skins on. Set the heads upright in an oiled baking dish. Spoon a little olive oil over them. Bake for 30 minutes or more, until the garlic is completely soft inside. To get the soft roasted garlic cloves out of the paper, wait for the heads to cool enough for safe handling, then hold the head by the bottom in one hand and use a spoon to help slide the cloves out of their paper skins. They should come out easily.

Serve with anything! Fresh salads, chopped veggies, cooked vegetables, vegetable chili, stir-fry, et cetera.

To make into a sauce: Blend several of the soft cloves with ½ cup olive oil and serve.

Arugula Pesto

This pesto makes a great sauce for dipping veggies or dressing salads. Substitute different greens for the arugula, such as fresh spinach or basil, and add fresh lemon juice (½–1/2 to 1 lemon).

- ½ cup extra-virgin olive oil
- 1½ cups arugula
- ¼ cup parsley
- 2 cloves garlic
- Sea salt

Blend all ingredients, adding a little water to achieve desired consistency. Add extra olive oil and a splash of vinegar to leftovers to make salad dressing!

Basil Pesto

- ½ cup extra-virgin olive oil
- 1½ cups chopped basil
- 2 cloves garlic
- ¼ cup pumpkin seeds
- Juice of ½ lemon or lime
- Sea salt to taste

Blend all ingredients, adjusting the ingredients to the desired consistency and flavor. Serve on fish or with veggies.

Mustard Dressing

- ¼ cup apple cider vinegar
- 1/3 cup olive oil, Udo's oil or flaxseed oil
- 1 tsp prepared mustard
- Dash sea salt
- Optional: 1 minced garlic clove; pinch of cayenne pepper or red pepper (omit if avoiding nightshade family)

Mix in large bowl or cup until blended.

Egg-, Soy-, Dairy-Free Mayonnaise

- 1 bunch curly-leaf parsley
- 1 bunch mixed scallions
- 4–8 big garlic cloves
- 1 lemon, juiced, or 2 Tbsp apple cider vinegar
- 1–1½ cups olive oil
- Sea salt to taste

Mix all ingredients together and blend (may add brown mustard to taste).

Horseradish Sauce

Makes enough for 3-4 good helpings of veggies

- 2 Tbsp ghee (omit during cleanse; can be included after cleanse)
- 1/3 cup olive oil
- 3 Tbsp freshly ground or prepared horseradish
- 3 Tbsp apple cider vinegar
- 1 Tbsp fresh dill or 1 tsp dried dill
- ¼ tsp sea salt
- Pepper to taste

Combine and warm all ingredients over low heat. Toss with steamed vegetables (leeks, brussels sprouts, carrots, etc.) and serve.

Guacamole

Avocados are okay after Digestive Cleanse.

- 2 avocados, peeled and coarsely chopped
- 1 small onion, coarsely chopped
- 1 tomato, chopped (omit if avoiding nightshade family)1–2 tsp fresh garlic, minced or pressed
- Juice of 1 freshly squeezed lemon
- ½–1 Tbsp fresh cilantro, chopped
- 1 tsp cumin
- Sea salt

Combine all ingredients and mash by hand or place in blender and blend until smooth. Serve with raw vegetables.

Raw Ranch Dressing

For Kidney and Liver Cleanses only
Yields 1½ cups
From www.choosingraw.com

- ¾ cups almonds, soaked overnight and rinsed
- 1 clove garlic
- ½ cup water
- 2 Tbsp lemon juice
- ¼ cup apple cider vinegar (a little more if you like it more tart)
- 3 Tbsp olive oil
- ¼–½ tsp salt
- ½ tsp dried thyme
- ½ tsp dried oregano
- ½ tsp onion powder
- 3 Tbsp fresh dill
- 3 Tbsp fresh parsley

Blend all ingredients in a high-speed blender, or blend all ingredients except for the oil in a food processor and drizzle the oil in until the mixture is creamy and emulsified. When dressing is blended, add a few more tablespoons of chopped herbs. Enjoy on top of a big green salad or with veggies.

Non-Ketogenic Dressing Recipes

Beet Dressing

Not ketogenic (too starchy)

- 2 medium-sized cooked beets (boil until soft ahead of time and remove the skins)
- ¼ cup olive oil
- 1 Tbsp stone-ground mustard
- ¼ cup apple cider vinegar
- ¼ tsp sea salt
- ¼ tsp freshly ground pepper

Combine all ingredients in a blender until smooth. For a sweeter taste, add more beets; for more "zip," add more vinegar. Dressing is thick.

Carrot-Ginger Dressing

From Peter J. D'Adamo's Eat Right 4 Your Type *cookbook*
Not ketogenic (too starchy)

- 2 medium carrots, chopped
- 1 Tbsp olive oil
- 1 1" piece fresh ginger, peeled
- 1 Tbsp fresh lemon juice
- Sea salt to taste

Place carrots, olive oil, ginger, and lemon juice in the food processor and pulse until a smooth consistency is reached. If the mixture is too thick, add water 1 Tbsp at a time. Salt to taste. Stores in the refrigerator for up to a week.

Drink Recipes

Green Drink

This is a staple of your cleanse! The green drink can take many forms:

- Blend leafy green veggies into your smoothie.
  - You may combine vegetables and fruits when they are liquefied, but avoid adding more than a few berries in order to promote fat burning and balance blood sugar. Avoid fruits altogether if your goal is ketosis.
- Freshly juice your own green vegetables like kale, parsley, or wheatgrass.
- Add liquid chlorophyll, spirulina, or a green drink powder (like Greens First Pro) to your beverage (water, tea, smoothie).

Star's Lemonade

Star's lemonade digests mucus, stimulates hydrochloric acid, and increases circulation. It is great for the sinuses and also supports the kidneys. It will help if you have a tendency to be "low energy."

- 1 lemon, juiced
- 10–12 oz warm or room-temperature water
- 1/10 tsp or more cayenne pepper 40,000 BTUs (optional since this is a nightshade vegetable)
- A little stevia, honey, or maple syrup is traditionally added, but this should typically be avoided during the cleanse

Stir well. Enjoy first thing upon rising.

Ginger Tea

From Shakta Kaur Khalsa's Kundalini Yoga

Immediately calming for the nerves and energizing to the body, ginger tea is good for everyone and especially helpful for women during their monthly menses.

- 4"–6⅛" thick slices of fresh ginger root (unpeeled is fine)
- 2 cups water
- Lemon juice

Bring water to boil and add ginger root slices. Boil until water is light brown in color, about 15 minutes.

Options:
- Add fresh lemon juice.
- After the cleanse, add stevia or honey to taste.
- Double or triple the recipe and keep in the refrigerator for continued enjoyment.

Herbal Teas

Any herbal (decaffeinated) tea is compatible with the cleanse. Mint, ginger, chamomile—are all supportive during the cleanse.

Enhance Your Water

You can enhance your water by adding:
- a slice of lemon
- a slice of lime
- a slice of cucumber
- up to 1 Tbsp apple cider vinegar in 8–16 oz water
- a splash of the Star's lemonade or ginger tea
- carbonation (via SodaStream, or purchase unflavored carbonated water)

Acknowledgments

There would be no book if I hadn't met the late Dr. Renee Welhouse. Dr. Renee devoted her life and career to helping others experience natural health and healing. I will forever be grateful to her and the staff of the Welhouse Center for opening my eyes and starting me on the path of natural healing. I also want to thank Michelle Jolly, Certified Health Coach, for her contributions to the book.

My friend Amy Walden showed an interest and helped me shape the book in its earliest stages, for which I am grateful. Thanks to Christie Mole and Beth Polen, who helped with editing and book layout. Thank you to my family members for your support in this endeavor.

Finally, thank you to the people of all ages who have given the Body Tune-Up a fair shake! Your positive experiences with the cleanse continually inspire me to share this information.

Appendix A: Organ Stress Chart

The signs on the following page are indicators of stressed organ systems and potentially indicate need for the cleanse for each section.

Signs of Colon Stress	Signs of Parasitic Infestations	Signs of Kidney Stress	Signs of Liver Stress

• Abdominal gas
 • Allergies
 • Arthritis
 • Asthma
 • Backaches
 • Bad breath
 • Chronic fatigue
 • Constipation
 • Depression
 • Diarrhea
 • Difficult weight loss
 • Distended abdomen
 • Food cravings
 • Frequent colds
 • Hemorrhoids
 • Holding on to grief
 • Hypertension
 • Hypoglycemia
 • Insomnia
 • Irritability
 • Prostate trouble
 • Skin problems
	• Absentmindedness
	 • Allergies
	 • Anemia
	 • Diarrhea
	 • Cravings for sweets
	 • Facial pallor
	 • Fretful sleep
	 • Itching (especially at night)
	 • General weakness
	 • Grinding teeth while asleep
	 • Joint or muscle pain
	 • Kidney problems
	 • Liver problems
	 • Mental dullness
	 • Severe fatigue
	 • Skin rashes
	 • Voracious appetite
		• Abnormal blood pressure
		 • Bad taste in mouth
		 • Bone problems
		 • Chronic low-back pain
		 • Ear infections & diseases
		 • Excessive fear & insecurity
		 • Fatigue
		 • Frequent urination
		 • Hair problems:
		   • loss
		   • premature graying
		   • split ends
		 • Hearing loss
		 • Incontinence
		 • Kidney stones
		 • Nausea
		 • Painful urination
		 • Premature aging
		 • Puffy face
		 • Reproductive imbalances
		 • Slow urination
		 • Swelling of ankles/legs
		 • Urinary tract infections
		 • Weight loss
			• Abnormal blood pressure
			 • Allergies
			 • Bad breath
			 • Bloating
			 • Brain fog
			 • Chemical sensitivities
			 • Coated tongue
			 • Constipation
			 • Dark circles under eyes
			 • Digestive problems
			 • Dizziness
			 • Eczema
			 • Emotional imbalances & repression
			 • Extreme body odor
			 • Eye problems
			 • Fatigue
			 • Gallstones
			 • Headaches & migraines
			 • Hypoglycemia
			 • High cholesterol
			 • Itchy skin
			 • Low blood sugar
			 • Lumps
			 • Menopausal discomfort
			 • Menstrual difficulties
			 • Mental confusion
			 • Muscle pain
			 • Swellings
			 • Vertigo

Appendix B: Left-Nostril Breathing

Left-nostril breathing not only helps promote healthy digestion and elimination, it also helps promote relaxation and sleep. Aim to practice three minutes daily.

Posture: Sit in a comfortable cross-legged position or in a chair with your spine straight and feet flat on the ground. Close your eyes if you choose. Tune in and center yourself.

Breath: Use the thumb of your right hand to block your right nostril. Inhale long and deep through your left nostril.

Mudra: The left hand is in giant mudra, with the index finger touching the thumb. The right thumb is blocking the right nostril and the other fingers are together, pointing straight up.

Time: 1–3 minutes.

End: Inhale deeply, hold your breath for 10–20 seconds, exhale. Repeat 2 more times.

Breathing through the left nostril stimulates the cooling, relaxing function of the body.

When you cannot sleep or need to reduce tension, breathe through the left nostril.

For long-standing issues with high blood pressure, this may be practiced for 10 minutes daily to help balance blood pressure, along with adjustments to your food plan.

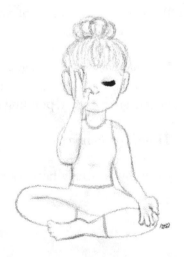

Appendix C: Compatible Supplements

Below is a list of the optional supplements that are especially compatible with the aims of the Body Tune-Up. You may want to plan ahead and consider purchasing them for your cleanse. Food is the foundation for your cleanse, and these supplements are optional. These supplements may be purchased at www.humannaturellc.com.

Ayur-Triphala by Douglas Labs—Useful for digestive issues, especially constipation. Take two up to three times daily as needed.

Baja Gold sea salt—The best available sea salt due to its high level and diversity of minerals. Celtic salt is a good close second.

Betaine and Pepsin by Ortho Molecular—This is a beet-derived supplement that helps support proper stomach-acid production. Do not take if you are taking steroids or have evidence of an ulcer. Contact a qualified health practitioner for guidance.

Body Tune-Up Critter Cleanse by Human Nature—Herbal blend in capsules taken during the Critter Cleanse.

Body Tune-Up Kidney Support by Human Nature—Blend of herbs and nutrients that support the Kidney Cleanse. Take two capsules with two meals daily.

Body Tune-Up Multistrain Probiotic by Human Nature—Adds good bacteria to the digestive system during the cleanse. Helps reduce cravings.

Body Tune-Up Liver Support by Human Nature—Tablets for the Liver Cleanse that help nourish the liver and promote Phases 1 and 2 detoxification. Take two tablets three times daily with meals. It is good to chew instead of just swallowing. Check with your physician before taking if you are taking prescription medications that affect blood pressure or the heart.

Digestive Enzymes by Allegany Nutrition—May be helpful in assisting the breakdown of food to nutrients. Helps alleviate digestive complaints and reduces food sensitivities. Try Allegany Nutrition AL-90 or AL-270. This is a good long-term supplement to take for complete digestion. Take two capsules with each meal.

G.I. Detox+ by Bio-Botanical Research—A capsule binder that may be used instead of the liquid bentonite. Start with two capsules daily and increase if desired, up to six per day. Take at least one hour away from food.

Glutagenics by Metagenics—For sensitive stomach and leaky gut issues. Take one heaping teaspoon in water before or after meals as needed for heartburn or acid reflux. Also may be used twice daily away from food to help overcome food sensitivities.

Green drink—Helps with detoxification, minerals, blood sugar control, and cravings and is an easy source of vegetables. Greens First Pro powder or chlorella tablets are popular choices.

Greens First PRO—A green drink powder (please review extensive ingredient list if you have food sensitivities). Add one scoop to eight ounces liquid.

Histo-X by Apex Energetics—A natural antihistamine supplement blend that includes butterbur and quercetin. Often very helpful for high-histamine issues. I suggest one or two capsules three or more times daily and reducing the dose as it's no longer needed.

ION* Biome by Biomic Sciences—Helps repair leaky gut and rebuild a healthy gut biome. Take one teaspoon three times daily before meals. This is a good long-term supplement to support a healthy gut.

Kidney Cleanse Tea by Hanna's Herb Shop—Dried herbs used in the Kidney Cleanse. Follow instructions in Chapter 9. Check with your physician before taking if you are taking prescription medications that affect blood pressure or the heart.

L-glutathione—Helps fix and prevent leaky gut and autoimmunity. Powerful anti-inflammatory/antioxidant. Assists with liver and cellular detoxification. Begin with one capsule daily with or without food or one teaspoon daily of a liquid.

Liquid bentonite (Sonne's #7)—Liquid clay that helps to gently detoxify the digestive system. It can cause constipation for some, so if you are prone to constipation, you may want to skip this. Another option is to take magnesium also to alleviate the constipation and get the detoxifying benefits of the bentonite simultaneously. Typically one tablespoon is taken with eight ounces of water at least one hour away from food in the Digestive Cleanse. This may be continued throughout the Body Tune-Up and beyond if desired.

Liquid chlorophyll—A liquid green supplement that can turn a beverage into a "green drink." Made from alfalfa. Look for brands without preservatives. Add one teaspoon or more to an eight-ounce beverage.

Mg-Zyme by Biotics Research—Blend of high-quality magnesium types. Useful for sleeping and constipation. Begin with one capsule at night before bed, then steadily increase dose until you are sleeping through the night and bowel movements are healthy. Too much magnesium may results in loose stools (you will no longer absorb it all and it will come out through the digestive system).

Multivitamin—Helps address nutrient deficiencies and supports detoxification. I suggest Ortho Molecular Alpha Base without iron, one with three meals, daily.

NAC (N-acetyl-L-cysteine) by Biotics Research—Helps to recycle glutathione and has many anti-inflammatory and detoxifying benefits. Take two capsules daily.

Natural D-Hist by Ortho Molecular or D-Hist Jr. for children—A natural anti-histamine blend including quercetin, nettles, NAC, and bioflavinoids. Often very helpful for histamine issues. I suggest one or two capsules three or more times daily.

Turmero by Apex Energetics—A liquid turmeric supplement that tastes delicious and carries all the benefits of this superfood in an easy-to-absorb formula. Adults, take one teaspoon one or two times daily with or without food.

Human Nature, LLC
Contact us if you'd like support on your health journey.
www.humannaturellc.com
Customer Support:
1-877-WELL-939 (toll free), 608-301-9961 (local)

Bibliography

Ajala, Olubukola, Patrick English, and Jonathan Pinkney. "Systematic Review and Meta-Analysis of Different Dietary Approaches to the Management of Type 2 Diabetes." *American Journal of Clinical Nutrition* 97, no. 3 (March 2013): 505–516. https://doi.org/10.3945/ajcn.112.042457.

Badger Mike. "Pasture and Feed Affect Broiler Carcass Nutrition." *APPPA (American Pastured Poultry Producers Association) Grit* 80 (March/April 2014). https://apppa.org/resources/Documents/Pasture%20and%20Feed%20Affect%20Broiler%20Carcass%20Nutrition%20--Final%20-%20rev%204-22-15.pdf.

Begley, Sharon. "Records Found in Dusty Basement Undermine Decades of Dietary Advice." *STAT* via *Scientific American*, April 19, 2017. http://scientificamerican.com/article/record-found-in-dusty-basement-undermine-decades-of-dietary-advice/.

Bischoff, Stephan C., Giovanni Barbara, Wim Buurman, Theo Ockhuizen, Jörg-Dieter Schulzke, Matteo Serino, Herbert Tilg, Alistair Watson, and Jerry M. Wells. "Intestinal Permeability—A New Target for Disease Prevention and Therapy." *BMC Gastroenterology* 14 (2014): 189. https://doi.org/10.1186/s12876-014-0189-7.

Bull, Matthew J., and Nigel T. Plummer. "Part 1: The Human Gut Microbiome in Health and Disease." *Integrative Medicine (Encinitas)* 13, no. 6 (December 2014): 17–22.

Carding, Simon, Kristin Verbeke, Daniel T. Vipond, Bernard M. Corfe, and Lauren J. Owen. "Dysbiosis of the Gut Microbiota in Disease." *Microbiology Ecology in Health and Disease* 26 (2015): 10.3402. https://doi.org/10.3402/mehd.v26.26191.

Clark, Hulda Regehr. *The Cure for all Cancers.* Chula Vista, CA: New Century Press, 1993.

Clemons, Zsofia, and Csaba Tóth. "Vitamin C and Disease: Insights from the Evolutionary Perspective." *Journal of Evolution and Health* 1, no. 1 (2016): article 13. https://doi.org/10.15310/2334-3591.1030.

Colbert, Don. *Dr. Colbert's Keto Zone Diet: Burn Fat, Balance Hormones, and Lose Weight.* Franklin, TN: Worthy Publishing, 2017.

Davis, William. *Wheat Belly: Lose the Wheat, Lose the Weight, and Find Your Path Back to Health.* New York: Rodale Books, 2011.

Haddad, Pierre S., Georges A. Azar, Simon Groom, and Michel Biovin. 2005. "Natural Health Products, Modulation of Immune Function and Prevention of Chronic Diseases." *Evidenced-Based Complementary Alternative Medicine* 2, no. 4 (December 2005): 513–520. https://doi.org/10.1093/ecam/neh125.

Hodges, Romilly E., and Deanna M. Minich. "Modulation of Metabolic Detoxification Pathways Using Foods and Food-Derived Components: A Scientific Review with Clinical Application." *Journal of Nutrition and Metabolism* 2015 (June 16, 2015): 760689. https://doi.org/10.1155/2015/760689.

Katzen, Mollie. *Vegetable Heaven: Over 200 Recipes for Uncommon Soups, Tasty Bites, Side-by-Side Dishes, and Too Many Desserts.* New York: Hyperion, 1997.

Khalsa, Dharma Singh, and Cameron Kauth. *Meditation as Medicine.* New York: Pocket Books, 2001.

Khalsa, Shakta Kaur. *Kundalini Yoga: As Taught by Yogi Bhajan: Unlock Your Inner Potential through Life-Changing Exercise.* New York: Dorling Kindersley Publishing, 2001.

Kharrazian, Datis. *Why Isn't My Brain Working?* Carlsbad, CA: Elephant Press, 2013. Illustrated edition.

Lemos da Luz, Protasio, Desiderio Favarato, Jose Rocha Faria-Neto Jr., Pedro Lemos, and Antonio Carlos Palandri Chagas. "High Ratio of Triglycerides to HDL-Cholesterol Predicts Extensive Coronary Disease." *Clinical Science* 64 (2008): 427–432. https://doi.org/10.1590/s1807-59322008000400003.

Lifestyle Matrix Center. *Pillars of GI Health In-Practice Guide.* LifestyleMatrix.com, 2018.

Maes, Michael, and Jean-Claude Leunis. "Normalization of Leaky Gut in Chronic Fatigue Syndrome (CFS) Is Accompanied by a Clinical Improvement: Effects of Age, Duration of Illness and the Translocation of LPS from Gram-Negative Bacteria." *Neuroendocrinology Letters* 29, no. 6 (December 2008): 902–910.

Maes, Michael, M. Kubera, and Jean-Claude Leunis. "The Gut-Brain Barrier in Major Depression: Intestinal Mucosal Dysfunction with an Increased Translocation of LPS from Gram-Negative Enterobacteria (Leaky Gut) Plays a Role in the Inflammatory Pathophysiology of Depression." *Neuroendocrinology Letters* 29, no. 1 (2008): 117–124.

Maintz, L., and N. Novak. "Histamine and Histamine Intolerance." *American Journal of Clinical Nutrition* 85, no. 5 (May 2007): 1185–96. https://doi.org/10.1093.ajcn/85.5.1185.

Manzel, Arndt, Dominik N. Muller, David A. Hafler, Susan E. Erdman, Ralf A. Linker, and Markus Kleinewietfeld. "Role of 'Western Diet' in Inflammatory Autoimmune Diseases." *Current Allergy Asthma Reports* 14, no. 1 (January 2014): 404. https://doi.org/10.1007/s11882-013-0404-6.

Mason, Paul. *From Fibre to the Microbiome: Low Carb Gut Health.* Video, July 11, 2018. https://www.youtube.com/watch?v=xqUO4P9ADI0.

Ohlgren, Scott. *How Health Works: The Advanced Cleansing Series.* Longmont, CO: Genetic Press, 2003.

Pitchford, Paul. *Healing with Whole Foods: Asian Traditions and Modern Nutrition.* 3rd ed. Berkeley, CA: North Atlantic Books, 2002.

Price, Weston A. *Nutrition and Physical Degeneration.* 8th ed. La Mesa, CA: Price-Pottenger Nutrition Foundation, 2008.

Sandek, Anja, Juergen Bauditz, Alexander Swidsinski, Sabine Buhner, Jutta Weber-Eibel, Stephan von Haehling, Wieland Schroedl, Tim Karhausen, Wolfram Doehner, Mathias Rauchhaus, Philip Poole-Wilson, Hans-Dieter Volk, Herbert Lochs, and Stefan D. Anker. "Altered Intestinal Function in Patients with Chronic Heart Failure." *Journal of the American College of Cardiology* 50, no. 16 (2007). https://doi.org/10.1016/j.jacc.2007.07.016.

Swiss Interest Group Histamine Intolerance (SIGHI). *SIGHI-Leaflet: Histamine Elimination Diet: Simplified Histamine Elimination Diet for Histamine Intolerance (DAO Degradation Disorder).* Version: October 16, 2015. https://www.histaminintoleranz.ch/downloads/SIGHI-Leaflet_HistamineEliminationDiet.pdf.

Tsai, Ming. *Blue Ginger: East Meets West Cooking with Ming Tsai.* New York: Clarkson Potter, 1999.

Vighi, G., F. Marcucci, L. Sensi, G. Di Cara, and F. Frati. "Allergy and the Gastrointestinal System." Supplement, *Clinical and Experimental Immunology* 153, no. S1 (September 2008): 3–6. https://doi.org/10.1111/j.1365-2249.2008.03713.x.

Yano, Jessica M., Kristie Yu, Gregory P. Donaldson, Gauri G. Shastri, Phoebe Ann, Liang Ma, Cathryn R. Nagler, Rustem F. Ismagilov, Sarkis K. Mazmanian, and Elaine Y. Hsiao. "Indigenous Bacteria from the Gut Microbiota Regulate Host Serotonin Biosynthesis." *Cell* 161, no. 2 (2015): 264–276. https://doi.org/10.1016/j.cell.2015.02.047.

CPSIA information can be obtained
at www.ICGtesting.com
Printed in the USA
JSHW040155210522
26120JS00005B/19